CHURCHILL'S POCKETBOOKS

Major Trauma

KT-430-804

Edited by

Adam Brooks FRCS(Gen Surg) DMCC
Consultant in Hepatobiliary and Emergency Surgery,
Nottingham University Hospitals NHS Trust, Queen's Medical
Centre Campus, Nottingham, NG7 2UH, United Kingdom

Lieutenant Colonel Peter F Mahoney
TD MSc FRCA FFARCSI FIMCRCSEd DMCC RAMC ADMEM
RCDM
Senior Lecturer Military Critical Care, Institute of Research
and Development, Birmingham Research Park, Vincent Drive,
Edgbaston, Birmingham, United Kingdom

Colonel Timothy J Hodgetts QHP MB
BS MMEd FRCP FRCSEd FFAEM FIMCRCSEd FRGS L/RAMC
ADMEM RCDM
Professor Emergency Medicine, Academic Department of
Military Emergency Medicine, Institute of Research and
Development, Birmingham Research Park, Vincent Drive,
Edgbaston, Birmingham, United Kingdom

Forewords by
C William Schwab and Ken Boffard

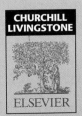

CHURCHILL
LIVINGSTONE

ELSEVIER

Edinburgh London New York Oxford
Philadelphia St Louis Sydney Toronto 2007

CHURCHILL
LIVINGSTONE
ELSEVIER

An Imprint of Elsevier Limited

© Elsevier Limited 2007. All rights reserved.

The right of Adam Brooks, Peter Mahoney and Timothy Hodgetts to be identified as authors of this work has been asserted by them in accordance with the Copyright, Designs and Patents Act 1988.

First published 2007

ISBN: 978-0-443-10255-4

British Library Cataloguing in Publication Data
A catalogue record for this book is available from the British Library

Library of Congress Cataloging in Publication Data
A catalog record for this book is available from the Library of Congress

Notice
Knowledge and best practice in this field are constantly changing. As new research and experience broaden our knowledge, changes in practice, treatment and drug therapy may become necessary or appropriate. Readers are advised to check the most current information provided (i) on procedures featured or (ii) by the manufacturer of each product to be administered, to verify the recommended dose or formula, the method and duration of administration, and contraindications. It is the responsibility of the practitioner, relying on their own experience and knowledge of the patient, to make diagnoses, to determine dosages and the best treatment for each individual patient, and to take all appropriate safety precautions. To the fullest extent of the law, neither the Publisher nor the Authors assume any liability for any injury and/or damage to persons or property arising out or related to any use of the material contained in this book.
The Publisher

ELSEVIER   your source for books,
journals and multimedia
in the health sciences

www.elsevierhealth.com

The
publisher's
policy is to use
paper manufactured
from sustainable forests

Printed in China

Major Trauma

For Elsevier:
Commissioning Editor: Timothy Horne
Project Development Manager: Lulu Stader
Project Manager: Kerrie-Anne Jarvis
Designer: Erik Bigland

CONTENTS

FOREWORDS

"Major Trauma", that which threatens life or limb, remains the leading cause of death for those under the age of forty and is rapidly becoming a daunting problem in third world nations as automobiles, industrialization and firearms emerge in these societies. Regardless of environment, military, civilian, urban, rural or austere, major trauma, if not quickly recognized, resuscitated and repaired, remains a challenge for all who practice in the emergency setting. These unpredictable and provocative medical events require a mastery of knowledge and proficiency of skill to assure competency and optimize outcomes. Maintaining these competencies is easy if one works within a busy emergency and accident unit or trauma center. However, most major injury does not initially present to these regional centers, but rather to smaller district hospitals or to emergency units that infrequently experience major trauma.

It is a privilege to introduce the **Pocketbook of Major Trauma** by Adam Brooks, Peter Mahoney and Tim Hodgetts. Each of these traumatologists are practicing clinicians and experts in their fields. This pocket sized book complements the major texts of traumatology by providing a portable manual of what to do in response to life threatening or major trauma. The editors are to be congratulated for selecting authors from around the world. Their clinical expertise at the beside or in the operating theaters translates to practical content that is honed by their experience and the editors have streamlined topics into the most pertinent clinical issues. The utility of this handbook is its clear and user-friendly layout with bolded axioms in the form of pitfalls and pearls, bulleted sentences and "at a glance" tables. In essence, the editors deliver a very useable manual that delivers contemporary well referenced material "short and sharp" and provides all readers a safe and effective way to manage major trauma, its physiologic consequences and anatomic dilemmas. It should be a companion of every physician, surgeon or house officer taking emergency call.

C. William Schwab MD FACS
Professor of Surgery
Chief, Traumatology and Surgical Critical Care
Department of Surgery
University of Pennsylvania School of Medicine
Philadelphia, Pennsylvania

In the ideal trauma world, in the ideal trauma environment, working within the ideal trauma protocols, the management of trauma would be straightforward and predictable. Life in reality is never that simple. Patients suffering from major injury often arrive in multiples, without warning, and without clearly defined injuries.

Good judgement comes from experience – Experience comes from bad judgement!

While there are many books detailing the management of trauma, many of them rely on science and previous experience. In many situations as a result of better primary (education to prevent the injury occurring) and secondary (design to minimize injury) trauma prevention, fewer people are being injured, and if injured, the injuries themselves may be less severe. The average Emergency Department outside of specialized Trauma Centres is, therefore, seeing fewer cases of major injury, and with the exception of military situations, many doctors lack experience in the management of penetrating injury, as well as the many pitfalls which can be discovered en route.

Tertiary trauma prevention implies that once the injury has happened, measures can be taken to minimize the effects of that injury. This book, written by authors experienced in both civilian (blunt and penetrating) and military trauma is designed to provide a straightforward, but detailed guide on what to do in most situations involving major injury and how to avoid the pitfalls of bad judgement. As importantly, the book provides clear advice on a 'fall-back position' - what do if the planned course of action doesn't work.

I regard it as a great honour to have been allowed to see this book before its publication, and hope that it will serve many doctors who have travelled beyond the limits of their judgement and will rely on others' experience.

Ken Boffard
Johannesburg
South Africa.

K D Boffard
Professor and Head
Department of Surgery
Johannesburg Hospital
University of the Witwatersrand,
Johannesburg, South Africa.

PREFACE

Churchill's Pocketbook of Major Trauma brings together current contemporary experience in the assessment, resuscitation and management of severely injured casualties from International Trauma Experts.

This includes the new UK Military trauma paradigm of '<C>ABC'; this is aimed at rapid management of catastrophic haemorrhage from ballistic injury, increasingly relevant to civilian trauma providers who may potentially manage victims of terrorist attacks.

The authors bring a depth of contemporary experience accrued from civilian trauma, recent terrorist incidents and the current military conflicts.

The aim has been to produce an easily accessible up-to-date pocketbook that will be of value to all trauma providers.

AB, PFM, TJH
December 2006

ACKNOWLEDGEMENTS

The editors wish to acknowledge the kind assistance of Mrs M Harris in providing administrative support for the project. All royalties and fees due to Lt Col Mahoney and Col Hodgetts from this project are being donated to a Military Charity.

CONTRIBUTORS

Roger A Band MD
Assistant Professor in Department of Emergency Medicine,
Hospital of the University of Pennsylvania, Philadelphia,
Pennsylvania, United States of America
Auto vs. pedestrian
Falls

Tracy R Bilski MD FACS
Assistant Medical Director ICU and Staff Trauma and General
Surgeon in National Naval Medical Center, Bethesda, Maryland,
United States of America
Blunt agonal resuscitation
Emergency department thoracotomy
Abdominal gunshot wounds

Colonel Mark W Bowyer MD FACS DMCC
Associate Professor of Surgery in Chief Division of Trauma and
Combat Surgery, The Norman M Rich Department of Surgery,
Uniformed Services University of the Health Sciences, Bethesda,
Maryland, Attending Trauma Surgeon, Washington Hospital
Center, Washington DC, United States of America
Blunt thoracic trauma
Shootings

Karim Brohi FRCS FRCA
Consultant in Trauma, Vascular & Critical Care Surgery in The
Royal London Hospital, London, United Kingdom
Peripheral vascular injury

Adam Brooks FRCS(Gen Surg) DMCC
Consultant in HPB Surgery, Emergency Surgery & Surgical Critical
Care in Nottingham University Hospitals NHS Trust, Queen's
Medical Centre, Nottingham, United Kingdom
Trauma teams
Catastrophic haemorrhage
Blunt agonal resuscitation
Emergency department thoracotomy
Austere and major incidents
Abdominal gunshot wounds

David Burris MD FACS DMCC COL MC USA
Professor and Chairman in The Norman M Rich Department of
Surgery, Military Region Chief ACS COT, Bethesda, Maryland,
United States of America
Explosions

Brendan G Carr MD MA
Department of Emergency Medicine in Division of Trauma and
Surgical Critical Care, Department of Surgery, The Robert Wood
Johnson Clinical Scholars Program, University of Pennsylvania
School of Medicine, United States of America
Maxillofacial injuries

Shamus R Carr MD
Staff Surgeon in US Naval Hospital Guam, Agana Heights,
Guam
Motor vehicle collisions
Motorcycle collisions

Ian Civil MBE OStJ ED FRACS FACS
Consultant Vascular and Trauma Surgeon in Auckland City
Hospital, Auckland, New Zealand
Overview of trauma epidemiology

Grant Christey BSc(Hons) MB ChB FRACS
Trauma and General Surgeon in Liverpool Hospital, University of
New South Wales, Australia
Tertiary survey
Impalement

Jim Connolly MBB FRCS(Ed) FRCS(Glas) FCEM
Consultant and Honorary Clinical Lecturer in Emergency
Medicine in Newcastle Acute Hospitals Trust,
Newcastle-upon-Tyne, United Kingdom
Soft tissue injuries
Trauma in pregnancy

Bryan A Cotton MD FACS
Assistant Professor of Surgery and Attending Surgeon in Division
of Trauma, Emergency General Surgery and Surgical Critical
Care, Vanderbilt University Medical Center, Director of Surgical
Critical Care, Nashville, Tennessee, Department of Surgery, Middle
Tennessee VA Medical Center, Nashville, Tennessee, United States
of America
Neck injury
Penetrating chest injury
Blunt abdominal trauma

Kate Curtis RN G.DipCrit Care MNurse(Hons) PhD
Clinical Nurse Consultant Trauma in St George Hospital, Sydney,
New South Wales, Australia
Scoring systems

Ben Davies MRCS(Eng)
Research Fellow in Cardiac Surgical Unit, Royal Children's
Hospital, Melbourne, Australia
Breathing

Scott D'Amours FRCS(C) FRACS(Gen Surg)
Consultant in Trauma Surgery, Emergency Surgery and General
Surgery, Liverpool Hospital, Sydney, Senior Lecturer in Surgery,
The University of New South Wales, Sydney, Australia
Abdominal stab wounds

Edward T Dickinson MD FACEP
Associate Professor in Department of Emergency Medicine,
Hospital of the University of Pennsylvania, University of
Pennsylvania School of Medicine, Philadelphia, Pennsylvania,
United States of America
Auto vs. pedestrian
Falls

Donovan Dwyer MB BCh DCH DipPEC FACEM
Specialist Emergency Physician Deputy Director of Trauma
Services in St George Hospital, Sydney, New South Wales,
Australia
Secondary survey

Angela S Earley MD LCDR MC USNR
Department of General Surgery in Naval Medical Center,
Portsmouth, Virginia, United States of America
Spine injury
Spinal cord injury

Susan Evans MD
Assistant Professor of Surgery in Carolinas Medical Center,
Department of Surgery, Charlotte, North Carolina, United States
of America
Cold injuries: hypothermia and frostbite
Obesity in trauma

Paola Fata MD FRCSC
Assistant Professor of Surgery in McGill University Health Centre,
Montreal, Canada
Circulation

Stephen C Gale MD
Assistant Professor of Surgery in Medical Director Surgical
Intensive Care Unit, Tulane University School of Medicine,
New Orleans, Louisiana, United States of America
Imaging triage in major trauma

Vicente H Gracias MD FACS FCCP
Associate Professor of Surgery in Medical Director Surgical
Critical Care, Hospital of the University of Pennsylvania,
Philadelphia, Pennsylvania, United States of America
Traumatic brain injury

Colonel Timothy J Hodgetts QHP MMEd FRCP FRCSEd FCEM
FIMCRCSEd L/RAMC
Honorary Professor of Emergency Medicine & Trauma, University
of Birmingham, Defence Consultant Adviser in Emergency
Medicine, Consultant Emergency Medicine, Royal Centre for
Defence Medicine, Birmingham, United Kingdom
Catastrophic haemorrhage
Austere and major incidents

James H Holmes IV MD
Assistant Professor of Surgery in Medical Director, Burn Center,
Wake Forest University School of Medicine, Winston-Salem,
North Carolina, United States of America
Burns

Jonathan A J Hyde BSc MB BS FRCS(CTh) MD
Consultant Cardiothoracic Surgeon in Sussex Cardiac Centre,
Royal Sussex County Hospital, Brighton, Tutor in Cardiothoracic
Surgery, The Royal College of Surgeons of England, United
Kingdom
Penetrating chest injury

Donald R Kauder MD FACS
Associate Director, Trauma Services in Riverside Regional Medical
Center, Newport News, Virginia, United States of America
Leading the team: preparation and establishing control of trauma

Patrick K Kim MD
Assistant Professor of Surgery in Division of Traumatology and
Surgical Critical Care, Department of Surgery, University of
Pennsylvania School of Medicine, Philadelphia, Pennsylvania,
United States of America
Damage control

Thomas Konig BSc (Hons) MB BS MRCS
Trauma Fellow, Royal London Hospital and Specialist Registrar
in General Surgery, Defence Medical Services in St Barts and the
Royal London Hospitals NHS Trust, London, United Kingdom
Trauma laparotomy

Lieutenant Colonel Peter F Mahoney TD MSc FRCA FFARCSI
FIMCRCSEd DMCC RAMC
Senior Lecturer in Critical Care, Royal Centre for Defence Medicine
Catastrophic haemorrhage
Anaesthesia and analgesia
Airway
Austere and major incidents

Francis Morris
Consultant in Emergency Medicine in Accident & Emergency
Department, Northern General Hospital, Sheffield, United
Kingdom
Ophthalmic injuries

Michael L Nance MD
Director, Pediatric Trauma Program in Josephine J and John
M Templeton Chair in Pediatric Trauma, Children's Hospital
of Philadelphia, Associate Professor of Surgery, University of
Pennsylvania School of Medicine, Philadelphia, Pennsylvania,
United States of America
Young patients—paediatric injury

Tarek Razek MD CM FRCS(c)
Department of Traumatology and Intensive Care in Montreal
General Hospital, Montreal, Canada
Circulation

Patrick Reilly MD
Associate Professor of Surgery in Vice Chief, Trauma and Surgical
Critical Care, Hospital of the University of Pennsylvania,
Philadelphia, Pennsylvania, United States of America
Spine injury
Spinal cord injury

Lt Col Rob Russell RAMC
Senior lecturer in Emergency Medicine Royal Centre for Defence
Medicine
Consultant and Lead Clinician in Emergency Department,
Peterborough Hospitals NHS Trust, Peterborough, United
Kingdom
Austere and major incidents

David W Scaff DO
Clinical Assistant Professor of Surgery in Penn State College
of Medicine, Trauma, Surgical Critical Care, General Surgery,
Lehigh Valley Hospital, Allentown, Pennsylvania, United States of
America
Trauma teams
Traumatic brain injury
Spine injury
Abdominal gunshot wounds
Injured elderly

C William Schwab II MD
Clinical Instructor of Urology in Eastern Virginia Medical School
Devine Tidewater Urology, Norfolk, Virginia, United States of
America
Genitourinary injury

Marianne Smethurst MB ChB MRCS(A&E)Ed
Emergency Medicine Specialist Registrar in Derbyshire Royal
Infirmary, Derby, United Kingdom
Care of infected and immunocompromised patients

Michael Sugrue MB BCh BAO MD FRCSI FRACS
Trauma Surgeon and Director of Trauma in Associate Professor
of Surgery, University of New South Wales Liverpool Hospital,
Sydney, Australia
Pelvic trauma

Nigel Tai FRCS
Consultant Vascular and Trauma Surgeon in The Royal London
Hospital, London, United Kingdom
Breathing

Caesar M Ursic MD FACS
Trauma Director in St Vincent Regional Medical Center, Sante
Fe, New Mexico, Trauma Medical Director, State of New Mexico,
United States of America
Scoring systems

Michael Walsh MS FRCS
Consultant Trauma and Vascular Surgeon in The Royal London
Hospital, London, United Kingdom
Trauma laparotomy

James L Williams FRCS (Tr + Orth)
Consultant Orthopaedic Surgeon in Taunton and Somerset
Hospital, Taunton, United Kingdom
Orthopaedic injury

Richard Wong She MHB (Hons) MB ChB FRACS (Plastics)
Consultant in Plastic, Reconstructive & Burn Surgery & Clinical
in Leader for the National Burn Centre, Middlemore Hospital,
Auckland, New Zealand
Burns

Dr Paul Wood FRCA
Consultant Anaesthetist in University Hospital Birmingham NHS
Trust, Birmingham, United Kingdom
Airway
Care of infected and immunocompromised patients
Anaesthesia and analgesia
Austere and major incidents
Trauma care of contaminated patients

CHAPTER 1

RESUSCITATION

LEADING THE TEAM: PREPARATION AND ESTABLISHING CONTROL OF TRAUMA RESUSCITATION AND OPERATING THEATRE

Background

A successful outcome in the management of the injured patient requires a thoughtful and organized approach to evaluation and treatment. This can be performed 'vertically' by a single provider using standard <C>ABC algorithms, or 'horizontally', by multiple care providers, modifying the approach so that many functions are being performed simultaneously (see The Trauma Team below). The horizontal method requires a team leader skilled in clinical resuscitation who, in addition, possesses leadership qualities and organizational skills. This chapter deals with the operational aspects of running a resuscitation, rather than on the clinical components.

PREPARING THE TEAM

Advance warning is a prerequisite for optimum team preparation. Knowledge of the clinical scenario before the patient arrives will allow more efficient use of personnel and resources.

History

- Penetrating or blunt mechanism
- Stable vs. unstable vital signs
- Interventions performed by emergency medical team (EMT)/ paramedics
  — cardiopulmonary resuscitation (CPR)
  — endotracheal intubation
  — needle chest decompression
  — intravenous (i.v.) access and volume infused

TRAUMA TEAM DYNAMICS

A successful trauma team must be well organized before the patient's arrival, and have an organizational structure that ensures success.

- Clear mission
  — each team member must have a clear understanding of the goals of the resuscitation
- Strategic plan
  — all team members must understand how the resuscitation will be carried out

- Organized role
  — each member must be assigned a unique role, and be well versed in what is required to accomplish the tasks that will be assigned
- Ownership
  — the team members must embrace their roles, and carry them out enthusiastically and competently
- Commitment
  — each team member must endorse the overall plan, and their role in the organizational structure
- Capacity/ability
  — each member must be fully capable of successfully carrying out his or her role
  — the team leader must thus assure that roles are assigned appropriately, and that all necessary equipment is available
- Trust
  — each member must trust that the other team members will carry out their assigned tasks, and that the leader will make the correct strategic decisions
  — the leader must trust that the team members will successfully carry out the assigned tasks and report clinical findings succinctly and accurately
- Leadership
  — there must be a strong, respected leader of the team, responsible for ensuring the team works as a unit to accomplish the mission

LEADERSHIP

The team leader takes on a difficult role, as they must make major clinical decisions, and communicate them effectively to a team that is operating under extremely stressful conditions. The successful team leader must be able to see the 'big picture' while controlling their own emotions.

Control yourself
- Don't panic
  — the team is looking to the leader to take control and direct them. A competent leader is well versed in the <C>ABC approach to care, and is able to improvise as needed
- Be systematic
  — following a logical sequence of thought and action informed by data collection and analysis will calm the team leader and the team

- Be a leader
  — voice: a command presence is enhanced by a commanding voice, loud enough to project over other speakers, but not screaming
  — this shows confidence without belittling the team
  — action: if the team seems to stall, or appears confused, stepping up to the bedside to assist and lead will set a positive example
  — calm: the more desperate the clinical situation, the calmer the leader must be. If the team perceives that the leader is out of control, chaos will ensue
  — know your limits: a leader is simply a leader, not a superhuman. The team will respect someone who is able to admit lack of knowledge or uncertainty, and who is willing to consult other team members or colleagues for their input
  — the best leaders are imbued with a number of unique leadership qualities:
    stamina: a leader who appears physically exhausted and/or emotionally drained will be ineffective in rallying the team to attend to the next trauma patient. Physical and emotional stamina are paramount, as are determination, a positive attitude and strength of spirit
    empathy: the effective leader must understand what each team member is experiencing, be it fear, indecision, anger, grief or elation. Furthermore, the successful leader must know the clinical capabilities of each team member, so that tasks can be assigned to persons with the appropriate skill level. Just as important is being attuned to the perceptions of the patient, and their fear, embarrassment, anxiety and physical pain. Showing sensitivity to team members and patients enhances credibility
    decisiveness: the best leaders are prepared to make life-or-death decisions in a matter of seconds with extremely limited information and, as importantly, be ultimately responsible for the outcome of those decisions. The trauma resuscitation unit is not the place for decisions by committee, the trauma resuscitation area is not the ideal venue to practise democracy

 The trauma resuscitation area is not the ideal venue to practise democracy

anticipation: the team should be well prepared for the arrival of a patient. Information gathered before arrival at hospital needs to be assessed by the team leader to ensure that roles appropriate to each team member's abilities are assigned, so that the sequence and flow of the evaluation can proceed calmly. This is especially important for patients known to be in extremis

credibility: the leader who is wrong too frequently, or who makes lame excuses for poor decisions, will not be a leader for long. Good team members won't follow poor decision-makers, but do want to know that their leader is willing to admit a mistake, take responsibility and move ahead

mentorship: when given the opportunity to berate a team member for making an error, the best team leader uses this as an occasion to teach and improve the skill set of the member. This creates a loyal ally and a skilled individual instead of an embarrassed and disgruntled adversary

Have a plan

- <C>ABC provides the framework upon which the team leader builds. The basics of initial assessment, and primary and secondary survey must be followed. One must be fully prepared for *every* clinical circumstance. There is no time to review the textbook when the patient is dying. The complexity of the patient's injuries within the context of the availability of medical resources will dictate variations in clinical care
- It is essential to communicate the plan of care on a frequent basis to all members of the team, and to assign a name to every task given
- Fight inertia—there is a tendency to alter the pace of evaluation and resuscitation based on the perception of the seriousness of the patient's injuries. This may cause delays in diagnosis and care
- Do not minimize physical findings or diagnostic information. Assume the worst and rule it out, and hope for the best

Control the environment

Trauma resuscitation rarely occurs in a private setting devoid of distractions. The team leader must be prepared to control the patient, the spectators, and the noise, all of which can interfere with concentration and divert attention away from the most critical issues at hand.

- The patient
  — an uncontrolled patient leads to an uncontrolled team. Do *not* let the patient assume the role of team leader, picking and choosing diagnostic and therapeutic modalities
  — it is extremely difficult to sort out whether an uncooperative patient is simply unpleasant, brain altered from injury or intoxication, or dying (or some combination!). Speaking with the patient and trying a brief period of negotiation may be helpful, but physical or chemical restraint should be considered early. If the patient continues to interfere with the flow of resuscitation, endotracheal intubation is always effective
- The crowd
  — the resuscitation of the most dramatically injured (e.g. impalement), or the presence of an intriguing social situation (e.g. law enforcement officer attacked) seems to attract crowds of well-meaning onlookers. Their presence can interfere with efficient movement and communication, and may become distracting to the team members. The leader must be at liberty to remove non-essential personnel from the area
- The noise: a number of factors can contribute to raising the noise level in the resuscitation area. The team members then raise their voices over the din, leading to a vicious circle of increasing volume and anxiety
  — background whispers: the crowd, as its members make quiet observations amongst themselves, can create a very loud background murmur
  — co-leaders: team members may seek to direct various phases of the resuscitation on their own. Such freelancing should be discouraged, as it adds to the noise and can lead to miscommunication among team members
  — irrelevant conversations: while it is a natural tendency to want to chat, all non-essential conversation between team members must by held to a minimum
  — the patient: the patient himself can contribute to the overall noise by asking questions, shouting to be heard, or screaming or moaning in pain. The team leader should designate someone to communicate with and reassure the patient, and ensure the provision of adequate analgesia. The combative patient will likely require endotracheal intubation

As one would re-boot a faulty computer, the noisy team must also be re-booted. This can be accomplished effectively by the team leader who, in a forceful commanding voice, calls out,

'STOP! EVERYONE QUIET!' In the ensuing silence, the leader can re-establish command and re-state the parameters for effective communication.

The noisy or distracted team may need to be 're-booted'
STOP ! EVERYONE QUIET !

Be flexible
- The patient, by means of anatomical injury, altered physiology and physical symptoms, will tell you what needs to be done—*listen*
- Listen to your team, and be prepared to admit you're wrong
- Be ready and willing to alter the direction of the initial resuscitation and care plans

THE TRAUMA TEAM

Background
- The traditional Advanced Trauma Life Support (ATLS)™ teaching is a systematic, vertical approach to trauma resuscitation based on a single provider (Fig. 1.1)
- The trauma team utilizes horizontal management based on multiple providers working in parallel (Fig. 1.2)
- Horizontal management
  — tasks are performed simultaneously by multiple team members
  — this is faster and more efficient

Organization
- See section on Leadership above
- Leadership with role allocation is central to an effective team (Fig. 1.3)
- Larger teams are not necessarily more efficient than smaller teams
- Team training through moulage (simulated casualty play) is valuable

Preparation
- Brief the team with available pre-hospital information
- Allocate team roles
- Ensure personal protective equipment (PPE) is worn
  — visor/goggles, face mask, gloves, lead apron, waterproof gown, tabard stating role (e.g. team leader)

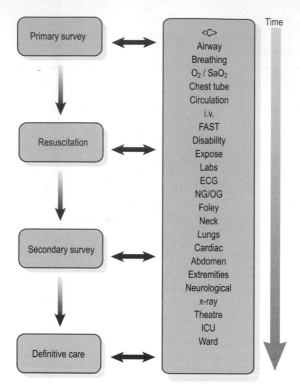

Figure 1.1 Vertical resuscitation: tasks are performed sequentially by a single provider. ECG, electrocardiograph; NG, nasogastric tube; OG, orogastric tube; ICU, intensive care unit

- Prepare equipment
  — airway equipment, i.v. access and fluids (± universal donor blood), procedure equipment (e.g. chest drain)
- Prepare drugs
  — analgesia
  — anaesthesia (e.g. for head injury with Glasgow coma score (GCS) ≤8)
- Prepare bed space
  — position staff for rapid transfer of patient to emergency department trolley
  — place chest x-ray (CXR) plate in trolley cassette

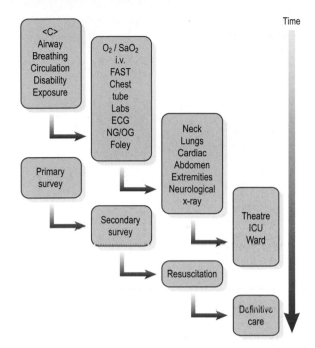

Figure 1.2 Horizontal resuscitation: tasks are performed by multiple team members, simultaneously reducing the total resuscitation time

Trauma team roles
- Team leader
  — controls and manages the resuscitation
  — consults specialists with regard to the management of specific injuries
  — makes critical decisions to prioritize further investigations and definitive treatment
  — generates the management plan
- Airway doctor
  — responsible for assessment and management of the airway: oxygen, airway adjuncts, endotracheal intubation
  — maintenance of cervical spine control where applicable
  — takes an initial history (allergies, medications, past illnesses/pregnancy, last meal, events/environment; AMPLE)

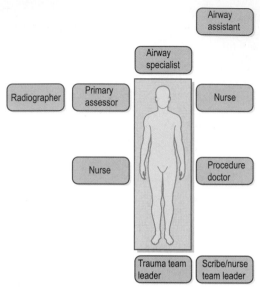

Figure 1.3 Positions of the trauma team members during resuscitation

- Primary survey
  — undertakes the primary survey from breathing (B) to exposure (E)
  — clinical findings are clearly spoken for team leader to hear and scribe to record
  — completes resuscitation paperwork
- Procedures
  — performs procedures depending on skill level and training i.v. access and blood sampling, chest tube, urinary catheter focused assessment with sonography for trauma (FAST)
- Nurse 1
  — applies monitors, assists anaesthetist with airway
- Nurse 2
  — removes clothes, assists with procedures
- Scribe
  — records team members present, history, vital signs observations, clinical findings and key decisions (with times)
- Radiographer
  — loads CXR plate before patient arrives
  — undertakes x-rays as indicated by the team leader

- Hospital specialists
  — undertake elements of the secondary survey at request of the team leader
  — undertake interventions if outside the competence of core team members (surgical airway, thoracotomy, venous cut down, diagnostic peritoneal lavage)

After the patient is transferred from the emergency department to theatres/intensive care unit (ICU)/ward the emergency department will reset to receive further casualties.

- Clean and restock trauma bay
- Return tabards and lead gowns to hangers
- Hot debrief by team leader if there are critical issues impinging on immediate effectiveness

Trauma team activation
- Criteria to activate the trauma team may be anatomical injury, changes in vital signs or the mechanism of injury (Table 1.1)
- 'Over triage' of up to 50% is acceptable to prevent the team not being activated for seriously injured patients ('under triage'): this is most common where reliance is on mechanism alone and can

TABLE 1.1 Trauma team activation criteria
Airway compromise
Signs of pneumothorax
Oxygen saturation <90%
Pulse >120/min or systolic BP <90 mmHg
Unconscious >5 min
An incident with five or more casualties
An incident involving fatality in the same compartment
High speed motor vehicle crash
Patient ejected from the vehicle
Knife wound groin or above
Any gunshot wound, mine or blast injury
Fall from >5 m
Child with altered consciousness and/or capillary refill >3 s and/or pulse >130/min
Child pedestrian or cyclist hit by a vehicle
Burns >10% child or >15% adult

be minimized by focusing on anatomical and/or physiological characteristics

CATASTROPHIC HAEMORRHAGE

Background
- In the pre-hospital setting a more aggressive use of tourniquets and the introduction of topical haemostatic agents has emerged as a policy of necessity within military medical services following the high level of blast and gunshot casualties in Iraq and Afghanistan
- First aid teaching has frowned on the use of tourniquets in civilian practice because of the fear of morbidity from inappropriate use, but their value in high energy traumatic amputations (blast) and in penetrating vascular injuries has been relearned in civilian terrorist incidents and military operational environments: they are a primary first aid intervention in these circumstances

<C>
- Rapid control of *catastrophic* external haemorrhage is the first priority in trauma care
  — it is the *<C>* of *<C>ABC*
- This can be achieved very quickly, allowing the resuscitator to move on to manage the *airway as per conventional trauma teaching*
  — if this is not achieved adequately in the pre-hospital phase then the patient is unlikely to survive to reach hospital
- Uncontrolled external haemorrhage is a common cause of avoidable trauma death (and the commonest cause on the battlefield)
- In hospital, consider the immediate use of uncrossmatched warmed blood and judicious use of recombinant Factor VIIa (**rFVIIa**) as part of **<C>**

External haemorrhage control
- Apply pressure to limb wounds and elevate the limb
- In catastrophic limb haemorrhage tourniquets save lives
- Topical haemostatic agents derived from volcanic rock and chitosan extract from shrimp shells have rapidly entered the military culture as a means to arrest catastrophic external haemorrhage, particularly in groin and axilla wounds not amenable to tourniquets

- The mechanisms of action of chitosan and volcanic rock extracts vary, but there is strong evidence of efficacy from animal models and human case series
- Tourniquet placed in an emergency **must** be reviewed as soon as possible to see if other means of haemorrhage control can be substituted

AIRWAY

Introduction
- The airway demands a high priority within <C>ABC to prevent early deaths from hypoxia
- A patent airway and adequate supplemental oxygen are fundamental principles of trauma resuscitation, irrespective of the mechanism of injury
- Airway management can be divided into basic, advanced and surgical techniques

Basic airway management
The majority of major trauma patients will be transported to the hospital supine on a spine board. In those with a decreased level of consciousness from head injury or drugs this will potentially jeopardize the integrity of the airway and may require advanced manoeuvres pre-hospital to secure the airway.

- Conscious patients with facial injuries (Le Fort fractures; destructive injuries of the jaw) may poorly tolerate lying flat. Those without risk of spinal injury should be initially managed sitting up or may choose to lie face down so the injured structures drop forward.

A stepwise approach to basic airway management can be taken:

Oxygen
- Oxygen is given to all self-ventilating patients who are victims of serious injury
- A non-rebreathing mask with integral reservoir bag is used
- High flow (10–15 l/min) to keep the reservoir partially inflated during ventilation will achieve an inspired oxygen concentration of around 85% (FiO_2 0.85)

Manual airway opening manoeuvres
- Jaw thrust
  — mandatory manoeuvre when there is suspected cervical spine injury
- Chin lift with head tilt

Simple adjuncts
- Oropharyngeal airways (OPA)
  — incorrectly sized OPA may induce laryngospasm and vomiting (if too long)
- Nasopharyngeal airways (NPA)
  — NPA is tolerated at a higher level of response and is effective when there is a degree of trismus (clenched teeth) in hypoxic patients, which prevents use of OPA
  — NPA has become many clinicians' first choice of simple adjunct
  — NPA is not free from risk
    basal skull fracture has been a traditional contraindication, but this is relative: an obstructed airway *must* be overcome and careful placement of NPA in patients with potential base of skull fracture is acceptable
    NPA can lead to haemorrhage when inserted brutally. To avoid this, use a lubricant and direct perpendicularly to the face: the nasal cavity is directed inwards, not upwards
  — NPA can be roughly sized as the tube with an internal diameter that just accommodates the patient's little finger
  — the correct sized OPA is the tube that best fits the distance between the corner of the mouth and the angle of the jaw

Advanced airway management
Progression to advanced techniques is necessary if

- Basic techniques fail to obtain a patent airway
- The airway remains at risk and must be protected
- There is a need to optimize ventilation by artificial means

Most patients with serious injury who require advanced airway management need an anaesthetic (such as ketamine or etomidate, which will not profoundly drop the blood pressure in a hypovolaemic patient) and a muscle relaxant (such as suxamethonium) to facilitate this.

- UK practice centres on an anaesthetist (or emergency physician) performing rapid sequence induction of anaesthesia (RSI)
- Injured patients who can be intubated without drugs generally have a poor survival although there are exceptions to this

Endotracheal intubation
- In-line manual immobilization must be maintained by an assistant during the entire intubation sequence if there is a potential cervical spine injury

- Preoxygenation via an anaesthetic circuit (bag–valve–mask apparatus)
  — the patient can either breathe spontaneously or be hand-ventilated
- A trained assistant applies cricoid pressure to minimize the possibility of aspiration of gastric contents
- The larynx is visualized by direct laryngoscopy
- The trachea is isolated with a cuffed endotracheal tube
- Every effort must be made to maximize success at the first attempt
  — including the use of a gum elastic bougie
- Tube position is confirmed
  — clinically (by listening for air entry)
  — detection of expired carbon dioxide (capnography or end-tidal CO_2 monitoring, performed with an electronic or disposable colorimetric sensor)

Surgical airway

In rare circumstances it is impossible to secure an airway by endotracheal intubation, usually because of upper airway and laryngeal distortion from direct injury or oedema.

> This is the 'Can't intubate, can't ventilate!' scenario

- When faced with this situation immediate access to the upper airway can be safely gained with minimal surgical expertise by a surgical cricothyroidotomy
  — initial preparation of the neck
  — define landmarks: thyroid cartilage and cricoid cartilage
  — transverse incision in the cricothyroid membrane
  — incision is dilated
  — insertion of tracheostomy tube (6.0) or endotracheal tube (care not to insert past carina)
- Purpose-designed commercial kits are available for surgical cricothyroidotomy
  — they share a common design to introduce a cuffed tube of appropriate length with an internal diameter ≥6.0 mm
  — the exact equipment used is less important than the absolute requirement to have core trauma team member(s) trained in the technique
- In situations of extremis a needle cricothyroidotomy permits translaryngeal *oxygenation*, but is inadequate for prolonged ventilation

— it is used only as a temporizing solution until a definitive surgical airway is established either at the cricothyroid level (surgical cricothyroidotomy) or by a formal tracheostomy

> If the skill and equipment is available for surgical cricothyroidotomy do not waste time with the needle technique

- A tracheostomy is fashioned at the level of the suprasternal notch
  — it is an elective procedure that requires surgical expertise, preparation and time

The airway with cervical spine injury

If a cervical spine injury is present or suspected none of the basic or advanced airway techniques is absolutely excluded:

- The airway always has primacy over the cervical spine
- Maintain integrity of the cervical spine through in-line immobilization
- Endotracheal intubation in the presence of a cervical spine injury is made more difficult by rigid in-line immobilization (spinal board, hard cervical collar and head blocks)
- Realistically it is foolhardy to attempt intubation with all these measures in place
- Remove the head blocks and unfasten (or remove the collar), *but retain manual in-line immobilization at all times*
- Laryngoscopy, Ensure a gum elastic bougie is at hand to railroad the tube
- The procedure can also be facilitated by selecting a smaller than normal size tube

The rules of airway management

1. Airway primacy. The airway is more important than the cervical spine. Think 'Big A with little c' (A–c)
2. No patient should be paralysed with neuromuscular blocking drugs unless the personnel and equipment standards can cope with the 'Can't intubate, can't ventilate!' scenario by needle or surgical cricothyroidotomy
3. Attempts at definitive airway management must not interfere with continuing oxygenation. Patients should not succumb to hypoxia during repeated misguided and failed attempts at intubation in lieu of bag–valve–mask ventilation. If expert help is required, get it early

4. Correct placement of an endotracheal tube or surgical airway should be confirmed by capnography. If in doubt, take it out
5. Be flexible with the 'rules' on airway sizes. The correct size is the one that does the job. In difficult situations be prepared to use smaller tubes
6. The management of the airway should not be accepted at handover unless the individual taking over the care is satisfied the techniques used are 'fit for purpose'.

AIRWAY INJURIES

The airway can be directly affected as a consequence of injury. The three most likely situations are

- Laryngeal or tracheal disruption from blunt or penetrating trauma
- Tracheal compression from a penetrating neck injury
- Airway obstruction from oedema following burns or smoke inhalation

Partial separation of the trachea requires careful assessment, particularly in respect to endotracheal intubation—if mishandled, this procedure may complete the disruption.

- A successful outcome may depend on available expertise in bronchoscopy and tracheostomy
- Vascular injury to the neck often needs a computed tomography (CT) scan to delineate the vessels involved
- Such patients should not be transferred for imaging until the airway is secured, as progressive compression may make later endotracheal intubation impossible

Burns oedema involving the soft tissues of the upper airway (in particular the tongue and epiglottis) is maximal between 12 and 18 h after injury.

- If there is any doubt regarding airway integrity, expert help should be sought early
- In severe cases the anaesthetist will 'gas the patient down' using inhalational anaesthesia
- The patient remains self-ventilating and the use of a muscle relaxant is avoided (see rule 2 above)
- When the patient is deeply anaesthetized direct laryngoscopy will be attempted
- In some centres the preferred approach is intubation using a fibreoptic laryngoscope in the awake patient

Equipment

Regular inspection and checking of equipment by nominated individuals is mandatory. This includes

- Anaesthetic machine (where used in the emergency department)
- Portable ventilator
- Suction
- Oxygen
- Bag–valve–mask apparatus
- Equipment and drugs for RSI
- Equipment for surgical airway

Summary

Hypoxia can be devastating and should not occur because of poor airway management.

BREATHING

Background

- 25% of all trauma deaths are due to chest trauma
- 90% of injuries can be managed with supplemental oxygen, good analgesia and a chest tube if appropriate
- The chest wall has anterior, posterior and lateral aspects

Maintain a high index of suspicion of thoracic trauma in:

- Patients who have sustained blunt head and pelvic/ lower limb trauma. (Think: what has been injured in between?)
- Patients who have sustained knife wounds to the neck or upper abdomen, or ballistic injury to any portion of the neck or torso

- The pleural cavity extends 2.5 cm above the medial third of the clavicle and, inferiorly, reaches the eighth rib in the midclavicular line anteriorly and the twelfth rib posteriorly (Fig. 1.4)

Assessment

Assessment, diagnosis and treatment of life-threatening thoracic trauma are carried out as soon as catastrophic haemorrhage is controlled, the airway has been secured and the cervical spine immobilized (initially by simple manual in-line stabilization if necessary).

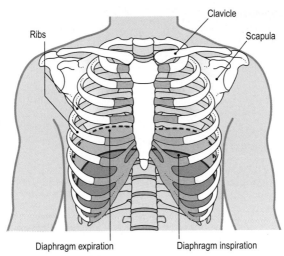

Figure 1.4 The extent of the thoracic cavity

- Oxygen should be administered via a high-flow mask (with integral reservoir bag) and a pulse oximeter saturation probe attached

  Proceed systematically with measured urgency, clearly announcing normal and abnormal findings as you go.
  The goal within the primary survey is to diagnose and treat the immediately life-threatening thoracic injuries. These are

- Tension pneumothorax
- Open pneumothorax
- Massive haemothorax
- Flail chest
- Cardiac tamponade may also be diagnosed at this time, but is considered a problem of circulation

  Signs of *blast lung* may be present early if the casualty was close to the point of an explosion.
  The presence of signs suggestive of thoracic injuries that, whilst not immediately life-threatening, may prove fatal unless confirmed will also be recognized during this assessment (Table 1.2).

- Inspection
  — check the patient's colour (normal/pale/ashen/cyanosed)

TABLE 1.2 Potentially life-threatening thoracic injuries		
Timescale of threat	Immediate threat to life	Delayed threat to life*
Diagnosis	Primary survey	Secondary survey
Conditions	Tension pneumothorax Open pneumothorax Massive haemothorax Flail chest Cardiac tamponade†	Pulmonary contusion Blunt cardiac injury Tracheobronchial injury Diaphragmatic rupture Oesophageal injury Traumatic disruption of the aorta
Investigations	Clinical skills +O_2 Saturations ±CXR	CXR 12-lead ECG CT FAST (pleural slide) Echocardiography Contrast radiology Bronchoscopy Oesophagoscopy (Flexible or rigid)
Management	Trauma team in emergency department	Specialist team after inpatient admission

*See section on definitive management of thoracic injuries
†See section on circulation

— is the patient lying comfortably or are they confused/
agitated/combative (always exclude hypoxia or shock before
attributing to intoxication)
— check for neck vein distension if not hidden by cervical collar
(marker of tension pneumothorax or cardiac tamponade,
*remembering that absence of vein distension does not rule out
either of these conditions*)
— rapidly assess respiratory rate and motion (depth/asymmetry/
paradoxical movements). These are best judged from the
end of the bed (especially if the patient is intubated and
ventilated, when paradoxical movements are less obvious)
— if there is blunt trauma, note bruises and patterns (seat belt,
steering column, tyre tracks)
— if there is penetrating trauma, note site/size/suction and
mark the wounds with paper clips for subsequent CXR
• Palpation
— thorax
actively feel for surgical emphysema, crepitus, painful areas
and displaced sections in front, around the sides and as far

       posteriorly as possible. Begin with hands placed either side
       of the sternum and work systematically
— neck
    if a cervical collar is applied, manually control the cervical
       spine and release the anterior part of the collar to allow
       examination
    (the cutaway in the collar may permit adequate examination
       in the primary survey so that the collar may be removed in
       the secondary survey)
    tracheal deviation is a late and infrequently observed sign
       of tension pneumothorax. Feel for laryngeal fracture or
       crepitus (evidence of a major airway injury)
- Percussion
  — this sign is difficult to rely on in a noisy trauma resuscitation
- Auscultation
  — assess the adequacy of air entry and added sounds in upper,
     mid and lower zones. Listen to the heart and determine the
     normality of heart sounds

- In penetrating trauma log roll *early* to exclude
  life-threatening injury on the back of the patient
- Always remember to examine the axillae

Immediate management: life-threatening 'B' problems

Tension pneumothorax (Fig. 1.5 and Table 1.3)
- Suspect in an agitated, dyspneic, tachycardic patient with
  overinflated hemithorax that moves little during respiration, ribs
  splayed apart, marked reduction of breath sounds and a
  hyper-resonant percussion note: all these signs indicate this
  injury
- Distended neck veins will not be seen if shocked from
  accompanying haemothorax or extrathoracic haemorrhage
- Tracheal shift away from the side of injury is a late sign and is
  likely to be followed by catastrophic drop in blood pressure and
  cardiac arrest secondary to loss of cardiac return

ACTION
- Do not wait for a CXR to confirm the diagnosis
- Needle decompression of the chest (needle thoracocentesis; see
  practical technique box) followed by insertion of an intercostal
  drain (ICD) is required (Table 1.4)

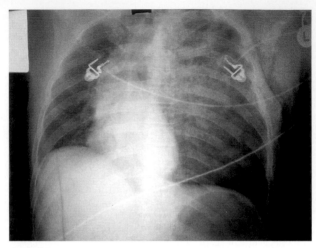

Figure 1.5 Tension pneumothorax. Arguably this chest x-ray should not have been taken (but in a trauma unit with rapid horizontal tasking and a pre-loaded chest plate it is understandable why it gets done)

How to perform a needle decompression
Equipment needed
- 14-gauge cannula
- 5 ml syringe filled with 3 ml of saline

Procedure
1. Locate medial and lateral endpoints of clavicle
2. Find midclavicular line
3. Locate convergence of midclavicular line and second intercostal space
4. Insert cannula/syringe through intercostal space, keeping perpendicular to skin, grazing upper border of third rib and aspirating on syringe
5. Stop once bubbles of air withdrawn. Disconnect syringe and listen for confirmatory hiss of expelled air and observe for rapid stabilization of patient's condition. Insert ICD
6. If no air aspirated, inject 1 ml of saline to flush any plug and reaspirate
7. If still no air, repeat with longer needle or move to fifth intercostal space on the midaxillary line

TABLE 1.3 Types of pneumothorax and their management

Type of pneumothorax	Simple pneumothorax	Open pneumothorax	Tension pneumothorax
Pathology	Breach in integrity of pleura leads to air in intrapleural space. Negative intrapleural pressure abolished Ipsilateral lung collapses	Ipsilateral lung collapses, and breach is sufficiently large to offer less resistance to movement of air than airway Air preferentially moves in and out of intrapleural space via breach rather than via trachea/bronchi	A flap-valve effect progressive accumulation of air in intrapleural space leads to positive intrapleural pressure, complete collapse of ipsilateral lung and displacement of mediastinum away from injured side Cardiac return is diminished
Signs			
Distress	Minimal	Notable	Marked
Respiratory rate	Normal or mildly ↑	↑	↑↑
Respiratory excursion	↓	Normal or ↓	↓↓
Percussion note	↑ Resonance	↑ Resonance	↑↑ Resonance
Auscultation	↓ Breath sounds	↓ Breath sounds	↓↓ Breath sounds
Treatment	ICD insertion after CXR	Occlusive dressing and ICD insertion	Immediate needle decompression and ICD insertion

CXR, chest x-ray; ICD, intercostal drain

- If needle decompression fails, immediately insert the ICD (see practical technique box)

How to insert an intercostal drain
Equipment needed
- 32- or 36-Fr chest tube with blunt flexible introducer (adult size) and underwater seal drain (or chest drain bag with integral flutter valve)
- Sterile gloves

TABLE 1.4 Trouble-shooting intercostal drain insertion		
Problem	Cause	Action
Cannot use fifth ICS, midaxillary line	Traumatized chest wall	Site ICD in anterosuperior or posterolateral plane
Finger sweep reveals adhesions	Pulmonary disease	If filmy adhesions, gently sweep away If fixed adhesions, reposition ICD at alternate site
Finger sweep reveals abdominal viscus	Diaphragmatic hernia	Gently sweep viscus away from drain track and insert drain. If any difficulty /resistance, abandon procedure: drain will be inserted at time of definitive repair
Drain not bubbling/swinging (check by asking patient to cough, or manually bag if intubated + ventilated)	ICD in lung fissure ICD in chest wall	Reposition drain, aiming more cephalad or basally so that track not in oblique fissure Remove and reinsert, ensuring that parietal pleura breached
Drain bubbling excessively	Bronchopleural fistula	Insertion of another ICD and refer for definitive treatment
Draining bile, urine, faeces	Concurrent abdominal injury	Laparotomy and definitive repair
Draining blood excessively	Massive haemothorax	Transfuse blood products whilst arranging urgent thoracotomy for definitive repair
ICD, intercostal drain; ICS, intercostal space; MAL, midaxillary line		

Equipment and procedure for injection of a chest drain

- 20 ml 1% lignocaine
- 20-ml syringe and Green needle
- Skin preparation solution
- Number 10 scalpel blade and handle
- Long haemostat forceps
- 0 nylon on a hand needle
- Adhesive tape and gauze dressings

Procedure
1. Ensure the patient is supine. Place their hand under their head (if practical) to get optimal access
2. Palpate and identify the fifth intercostal space and trace laterally until the midaxillary line is encountered. Mark a spot 1 cm anterior to this point
3. Prep the skin. Infiltrate 20 ml of lignocaine 1% at this site. The initial 10 ml should be used to raise a large skin weal. The needle should then be advanced in a track that grazes the top of the sixth rib, infiltrating down to the sensitive parietal pleura. This may also be supplemented with intercostal nerve blocks
4. Fill the underwater seal drain with the correct amount of saline (where used rather than a chest drain bag) and set up the sterile trolley with the sterile field, chest tube, haemostat, skin prep and 0 nylon. Insert the blunt introducer into a distal hole of the chest tube; where a chest drain bag is used connect this now (the drain will function immediately on insertion and there will be no blood spilled on the floor). If a sharp trocar is supplied with the chest tube, remove and discard it
5. Make a 2.5 cm skin incision over the weal of lignocaine, parallel to the rib. Deepen the incision through the subcutaneous fat and superficial fascia. Swap the scalpel for the long haemostat and use a muscle-splitting approach to track bluntly down through the intercostal muscles to the pleura
6. Bluntly pierce the pleura with the haemostat. This part is frequently very painful. Systemic opioids (e.g. 2–5 mg i.v. morphine) or ketamine (up to 0.5 mg/kg i.v.) given prior to starting the procedure will reduce the pain. A hiss of air or gush of blood usually accompanies perforation of the pleura
7. Insert a finger into the pleural cavity to confirm entry and perform finger sweep, feeling for lung and adhesions
8. Insert the chest drain with the flexible introducer, directing the tube posteriorly and towards the opposite shoulder. Remove the flexible introducer and push the drain in
9. Connect to the underwater seal drain (or drainage bag), and ensure draining/swinging/bubbling (see Troubleshooting chest drains)

> 10. Secure to skin with 0 suture, augmented by dressing
> and adhesive tape. Request CXR

- Reassess, continue the primary survey and take a CXR

> ⚠️ Be wary of the potential for repeat tension in patients
> who have undergone chest decompression in the field.
> The cannula may be malpositioned, plugged or displaced

Open pneumothorax
- Suspect in any chest wound/defect that bubbles and/or sucks as
  the patient breathes in and out
- This may have been treated in the field with an Asherman™
  chest seal or square dressing left untaped down one side (the
  latter improvised technique is suboptimal)

ACTION

- Immediately site an ICD on the same side as the injury, remote
  from the injury itself
- Place an occlusive dressing (Opsite™, Tegaderm™) over the
  wound
- Arrange lavage and definitive repair of the defect in theatre

Massive haemothorax (Fig. 1.6 and Table 1.5)
- Clinical examination is a blunt diagnostic tool: CXR or portable
  ultrasound examination are essential parts of the primary survey
- Key diagnostic features are reduced chest wall excursion, stony
  dull percussion note, and diminished breath sounds in a shocked
  patient
- CXR reveals 'white-out' of the affected side

ACTION

- Initial treatment is to ensure adequate i.v. access via two 14-G
  cannulae, followed by insertion of an ICD. This will reduce
  the shunt, allow assessment of the amount of haemorrhage,
  and reduce the likelihood of complications (chest infection,
  empyema, restrictive fibrous cortex)
- Urgent thoracotomy is required if >1500 ml of blood drains
  immediately or if >200 ml/h is drained for >4 h. However, there
  is no obligation to wait for these thresholds to be reached before
  proceeding to surgery in a shocked patient with severe thoracic
  haemorrhage

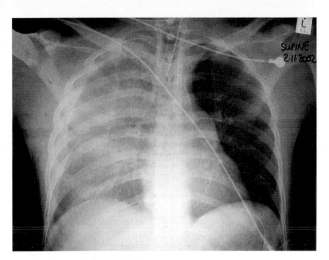

Figure 1.6 Massive haemothorax

TABLE 1.5 Causes of massive haemothorax		
Region	*Structure*	*Comments*
Chest wall	Intercostal vessel Internal mammary artery Multiple fractured ribs	Responsible for majority of haemothoraces
Lung	Parenchyma Segmental/lobar vessels	Lung expansion will tamponade bleeding
Mediastinal vasculature	Superior/inferior vena cavae Aorta Innominate vessels Carotid artery Subclavian vessels Hilar vessels/pulmonary artery or vein	Damage to large calibre, high pressure vessels likely to cause rapid haemorrhage and death
Heart	Right heart structures Left heart structures	Not a frequent cause of haemothorax in patients who survive to reach hospital
Intra-abdominal	Solid organs Hollow organs Blood vessels	Suspect from missile/stab trajectory, wound pattern, abdominal signs of bleeding

- Do not clamp the drain. There is no evidence that clamping the drain as a temporizing manoeuvre improves outcome
- Obtain a post insertion CXR to confirm position of ICD

- **Do not rely on chest drainage volumes as an accurate reflection of ongoing haemorrhage**
- **Drains can easily become blocked. Serial CXR is a useful adjunct in this regard**

Flail chest (Fig.1.7)
- Arises when three or more ribs are fractured segmentally. The resultant 'island' of discontinuous chest wall can no longer take part in effective ventilation
- Associated with severe underlying pulmonary contusion (the prime cause of subsequent respiratory failure), haemothorax and pneumothorax
- Characteristic paradoxical motion of flail segment—inwards during inspiration, outwards during expiration—may not be present if the patient is ventilated or if there is muscular splinting secondary to pain (latter in conscious patients only)

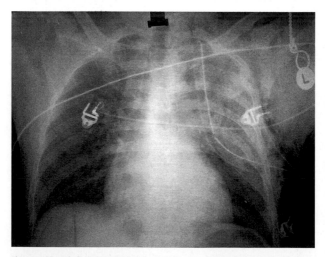

Figure 1.7 Left flail chest with associated upper lobe pulmonary contusion. A chest drain has been placed because of suspicion of associated pneumothorax (note surgical emphysema) and to enable intrapleural delivery of local anaesthesia

ACTION

- Supplemental oxygen and adequate analgesia are essential
- Pain relief should initially be i.v. morphine (10 mg in 10 ml normal saline, 2–4 mg boluses titrated to pain)
- Subsequent analgesia options include
  — epidural analgesia
  — patient-controlled analgesia
  — intercostal nerve blockade
  — pleural block (lignocaine/marcaine mixture instilled via chest tube)
- Observe closely for signs of progressive respiratory depression in high dependency/critical care setting
- Early intubation and ventilation is advocated, particularly if:
  — respiratory rate >35/min
  — oxygen saturation <90% on 15 l/min oxygen therapy
  — rising PCO_2 on serial arterial blood gases
- Non-invasive ventilation (continuous positive airway pressure) may be useful in a subset of patients who do not require invasive ventilation, but who are at high risk of deterioration

CIRCULATION

Background

Unrecognized or inadequately treated haemorrhage remains a significant cause of death from major trauma. Once <C>catastrophic haemorrhage is addressed the next phase of circulation is the recognition of concealed haemorrhage

- Loss of circulating blood volume can occur externally or internally
- Concealed haemorrhage should be actively considered in trauma patients

Concealed haemorrhage recognition

Massive internal blood loss can occur from four sites:

- Thorax
  — each hemithorax can accommodate several litres of blood
  — a massive haemothorax occurs when >1500 ml is contained within a hemithorax
  — *exclude by clinical examination and CXR*

- Abdomen
  — in blunt trauma this is usually from solid organ injury
  — do not be misled into thinking that an undistended abdomen does not contain blood
  — *exclude by clinical examination and FAST (or CT or diagnostic peritoneal lavage; DPL)*
- Pelvis and retroperitoneum
  — the retroperitoneum is a space that can potentially accommodate a volume of 2000 ml
  — in the presence of an *open book* pelvic fracture (where the pubic symphysis is widened >2 cm) this space can increase to accommodate 6000 ml
  — *exclude by pelvis x-ray and assessment of urine for macroscopic/microscopic haematuria (and CT in specific cases)*
- Orthopaedic injuries
  — one-third or more of a trauma victim's blood volume can be lost around a femur fracture
  — *exclude by clinical examination and limb x-ray*

Clinical and laboratory findings

- Lactate, base deficit and coagulopathy are useful indicators of severe injury and the patient's response to resuscitation
- However, beware of the following
  — changes in blood pressure and heart rate do not reliably indicate the extent of haemorrhage
  — young trauma patients can maintain their blood pressure for a sustained period and demonstrate little increase in heart rate until they dramatically decompensate
  — haemoglobin and haematocrit will not reliably measure the amount of blood loss, particularly if the patient presents shortly after injury

Resuscitation

- <C>ABC priorities are addressed simultaneously within a horizontal team-based approach to trauma resuscitation
- Catastrophic external haemorrhage is arrested as it is seen, although will be unusual in those that survive to reach hospital
- A secure airway and effective gas exchange is a parallel priority

Fluid resuscitation

- Target systolic blood pressure is 100 mmHg in adults
- Crystalloid is the preferred initial fluid if blood products are not readily available or are needed immediately

Vascular access
- A 14-gauge cannula in each antecubital fossa is the traditional teaching, although current guidelines for fluid resuscitation advocate more judicious infusion than that advocated in the 1980s and 90s of 2 l crystalloid given rapidly and routinely
- Femoral vein access should be used when the upper extremity route is not possible (percutaneous, or cutdown onto the saphenofemoral junction)
- Skilled providers can place an 8.5 rapid infusion line into the internal jugular vein, the subclavian vein or the femoral vein

- Boluses of 250 ml are given, with assessment for effect after each bolus
- For those with persistent signs of haemorrhage (no response or transient response to fluid resuscitation), blood transfusion must be considered when crystalloid infusion exceeds 30 ml/kg (2–3 l crystalloid in an average 70 kg adult)
- Uncrossmatched, type O packed red blood cells should be used in the patient with exsanguinating haemorrhage (O Rh-neg in females; O Rh-neg or O Rh-pos in males)
- Type-specific blood should be substituted as soon as it is available
- In life-threatening haemorrhage, transfusion will have no effect if the primary injuries are not adequately addressed:
  — *thorax*. If >1500 ml is drained after chest tube insertion, surgery will be needed
  — *abdomen*. Free fluid on FAST or grossly positive DPL warrants surgery
  — *pelvis*. Stabilize the pelvic ring by wrapping with a bed sheet, or commercial pelvic splint. Angiographic embolization may be required
  — *limb fractures*. These should be splinted. A femur fracture requires traction, which can be rapidly applied using a commercial splint
- Massive transfusion for life-threatening haemorrhage will result in
  — hypothermia
  — acidosis
  — coagulopathy
- The presence of hypothermia, coagulopathy and acidosis is termed the *lethal triad*

Hypothermia

- Hypothermia is defined as a core temperature <35°C
- The greatest potential for heat loss is massive fluid resuscitation *so warm the fluid*
- Mortality increases significantly for trauma patients with a core temperature of <34°C and approaches 100% if the core temperature falls below 32°C
- Effects of hypothermia are
  - ↓heart rate and ↓cardiac output
  - ↑systemic vascular resistance and dysrhythmias
  - central nervous system depression
  - ↓glomerular filtration rate and sodium reabsorption
  - coagulopathy (platelet dysfunction and sequestration)

Acidosis

- Effects of acidosis are
  - ↓myocardial contractility
  - ↓inotropic response to catecholamines
  - ventricular dysrhythmias
  - rate of activated Factor X formation by activated Factor VII/tissue factor is substantially reduced if pH<7.4
  - may cause disseminated intravascular coagulation and consumptive coagulopathy

Coagulopathy

- Remember that primary trauma resuscitation fluids such as crystalloids and packed red blood cells do not contain coagulation factors
- Tissue factor exposure secondary to trauma results in activation of the coagulation cascade and consumption of clotting factors
- The effects of dilution and hypothermia are additive
- Current (2006) US Military resuscitation policy at the Combat Support Hospital in Baghdad is to give fresh thawed plasma very early in the resuscitation and continue to give it in a 1:1 ratio with packed cells in the severely injured patient

Avoiding the lethal triad during massive transfusion

- Raise the temperature in the resuscitation and operating rooms
- Give fluids from a warming cabinet or administer through Level I infuser (delivers fluids at a maximum temperature of 41°C)
- Ventilator circuits should be warmed
- Avoid hypoventilation and excessive saline use, as this will worsen acidosis
- Apply a warm air blanket covering all exposed areas

- Use principles of damage-control surgery and abbreviate surgical interventions once haemorrhage control has been achieved, before the development of irreversible physiological endpoints

Use of clotting factors in massive haemorrhage

- Give early consideration to replacing clotting factors using fresh frozen plasma, platelets and cryoprecipitate in massively haemorrhaging patients
- Use of empirical strategies include
  - 1 unit of fresh frozen plasma for every 4–6 units of packed red blood cells or 2 units of fresh frozen plasma based on prothrombin time >18 s
  - use of 1:1 fresh frozen plasma to every unit of packed red cells within contemporary injured US military population
- Evidence for use of this first strategy is based on elective surgery patients who are euvolaemic—trauma patients are volume-contracted as a result of haemorrhage, therefore for the same volume of bleeding the degree of factor loss is greater
- In addition, volume resuscitation with crystalloid and packed red blood cells further dilutes plasma coagulation factors
- *Adopt an aggressive coagulation factor transfusion strategy to avoid dilutional coagulopathy following traumatic haemorrhage*

Use of recombinant factor viia in massive haemorrhage

- rFVIIa (NovoSeven® Novo Nordisk A/S, Bagsværd, Denmark) has been used 'off-label' in trauma to control life-threatening traumatic bleeding that has been uncorrected by other means. Despite favourable anecdotal, animal modelling, short-case series and phase II clinical trial evidence rFVIIa is not currently licensed for use in trauma patients
- rFVIIa amplifies coagulation at the local site of injury where tissue factor and phospholipids are exposed
- rFVIIa accelerates the tissue factor-dependent pathway and generates a thrombin burst along with platelet surface interactions
- Results from an international phase II study indicate no excess of critical complications and a reduction in the consumption of blood products
- The more common dosing for acute traumatic haemorrhage is 50–100 μg/kg

The management of patients with massive transfusion requirements is summarized in Fig. 1.8.

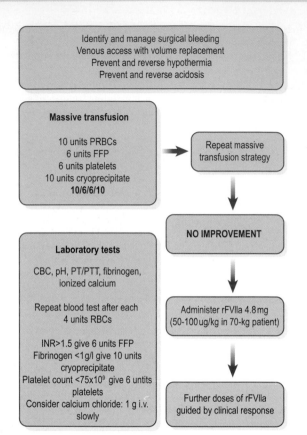

Figure 1.8 Management of patients with massive transfusion requirement. PRBC, Packed red blood cells; FFP, fresh frozen plasma; CBC, complete blood count; PT/PTT prothrombin time/partial thromboplastin time; INR, international normalized ratio

FURTHER READING

Boffard K D, Riou B, Warren B et al 2005 Recombinant factor VIIa as adjunctive therapy for bleeding control in severely injured trauma patients: two parallel randomized, placebo-controlled, double blind clinical trials. Journal of Trauma 59(1):8–15

Mattox K L, Moore E E, Feliciano D V 2004 Bleeding and coagulation complications, trauma, 5th edn. McGraw–Hill, New York

BLUNT AGONAL RESUSCITATION

Background
- Patients who arrive in extremis (death within minutes without intervention) present diagnostic and treatment dilemmas that demand immediate critical management decisions
- In penetrating injury the trajectory of the projectile or the organ system injured can be deduced by clinical evidence (although this is not wholly reliable)
- In blunt trauma there are at least three major body cavities (thorax, abdomen and pelvis) that can hide significant injury, and these must be investigated to determine injury, feasibility of repair and patient salvage

> The blunt trauma patient without measurable pre-hospital vital signs or signs of life is 'dead on arrival' and no resuscitation attempts should be made

Triage of the body cavities
A patient who arrives in the emergency department in extremis should undergo the following procedures

- Control of external catastrophic haemorrhage
- Obtain a definitive airway (done in parallel to control of haemorrhage)
- Obtain intravenous access and infuse crystalloid and uncrossmatched blood
- Thoracic cavity triage: place bilateral chest tubes
  — if >1500 ml initial output from either chest tube or ongoing haemorrhage from chest tubes, move to the operating room
- Abdominal cavity triage: FAST or DPL
  — if grossly positive, move to the operating room
- Pelvic cavity triage: pelvic x-ray
  — if the pelvis is unstable, place a stabilization device (Circumferential Sheet; Trauma Pelvic Orthotic Device™ [TPOD]; SAM splint)

SECONDARY SURVEY

Background
The secondary survey is a comprehensive examination of the injured patient. A systematic approach should be adopted from head to toe, and injuries recorded as they are discovered.

The management, organization of specialist consultations and investigation of injuries discovered in the secondary survey should be undertaken after life- and limb-threatening issues have been resolved.

Further detail on specific injuries/management can be found in the specific chapters in the specialist sections.

HEAD

SCALP

- Examine the entire scalp for laceration, bogginess, contusion and fracture
- Often neglected in primary survey as a site for significant bleeding
- Suture early, particularly in children, the elderly, coagulopathic patients and those with compound fractures
- Stapling is a rapid option and does not interfere with CT images

- The bleeding scalp can be a source of significant haemorrhage
- Suture early, pressure dress and closely monitor for ongoing bleeding

Eyes

- Periorbital structures
- Periorbital haematomas = orbital rim fracture or 'blow out' orbital fractures until proven otherwise
  — palpate orbital rim for step or tenderness
    tenderness over the inferior and/or lateral aspect of the orbital rim suggests zygomatic fracture or Le Forte type fractures
    absence of tenderness suggests orbital floor or medial wall fracture secondary to direct globe trauma
    direct blunt globe trauma—orbital floor and wall more likely to fracture (blow out) than globe rupture

 A 'black eye' can be a late sign of orbital floor or medial wall fracture

Signs of orbital floor/blow out fracture
- unilateral epistaxis
- infraorbital nerve neuropraxia
- diplopia secondary to extraocular muscle entrapment

> lid laceration—if the margin, muscle, punctum, canaliculus or lacrimal gland is involved or orbital fat is visible, call for an ophthalmology consult
>
> eye assessment is often neglected because of eyelid swelling and inaccessibility

Local anaesthetic and paper clip lid retraction allows globe assessment

Look for

- Visual acuity—the vital sign of the eye
- Perilimbic haematoma
- Eccentric pupil = globe rupture until proved otherwise
  - avoid further globe pressure
  - apply shield
  - i.v. antibiotics
  - urgent eye review
- Pupillary response
  - dilated = raised intracranial pressure (ICP)
    ischaemic/hypoxic brain injury
    traumatic mydriasis (not a systemic atropine affect)
  - constricted = opiates
    brainstem pathology
- Lens: confirm presence and remove contact lens

Remove contact lenses

- Systemic (i.v.) atropine does not cause dilated pupils in standard dose: look for another cause
- Neuromuscular paralysis in the intubated patient does not affect pupillary signs, as this is an autonomic function

Nose
- Examine for cerebrospinal fluid (CSF) leak
  - 'ring' sign on paper
- Simple fracture is common, but may be part of a medial orbital wall fracture (nasorbitoethmoid (NOE) complex), or complex facial fractures of the Le Forte type (see below: Maxillofacial)
  - consider facial CT

- Examine for septal haematoma
  — needs semiurgent evacuation to avoid cartilaginous septal resorption

Mouth
- Lip lacerations
  — vermilion border involvement requires excellent apposition for good cosmetic outcome
- Through and through lacerations
  — look closely for retained foreign body—teeth!
- Mucosal and tongue lacerations
  — suture with silk or dissolvable materials if >1.5 cm
  — warn of likely tongue deformity (retraction) at laceration site
  — penicillin antibiotic prophylaxis
- Facial lacerations
  — look for muscle, cranial nerve, parotid duct involvement
- If intraoral examination reveals bleeding from the parotid duct, the facial nerve must be injured as well
  — urgent specialist review

Teeth
- Avulsed teeth need replacement within the hour for good outcome
  — % tooth survival decreases by 1% for every minute not in the socket
- Fractured teeth
  — if pulp visible, dental review is necessary *as soon as possible* (<24 h)
  — for analgesia and to ensure tooth viability, use calcium hydroxide paste with glass ionomer cement

Initial dental care is cheap, easy and saves the patient thousands of pounds

Ears
- Pinna
  — simple lacerations can be sutured
    warn of skin retraction and deformity around the edges
  — perichondrial haematomas
    need early evacuation to avoid cartilage degeneration and ear deformity ('cauliflower ear')
    techniques include incision and drainage or needle aspiration followed by petroleum gel gauze compression bandaging

- External auditory meatus
  — haemotympanum suggests base of skull fracture
  — ruptured haemotympanum suggests penetrating trauma or barotrauma (explosions)

Maxillofacial

- Maxillary fractures
  — check for midface mobility
- Mandibular fractures
  — tenderness, interdental bleeding, trismus, subjective malocclusion are suggestive of fracture
- Condylar fractures
  — assess condyles for fracture and/or dislocation by a little finger inserted into the anterior part of external auditory meatus whilst patient opens and closes mouth

---

- Severe midface and mandibular fractures invariably threaten the airway and may become a source of major blood loss—intubate early
- Blood loss can be monitored and stemmed by orogastric tube placement and posterior pharyngeal packing, respectively
- Maxillofacial fracture reduction and/or embolization may need consideration if bleeding is ongoing

---

NECK

- Maintain in-line stabilization whilst releasing collar to assess neck formally

---

- **Beware penetrating neck injury: prepare for imminent airway loss and rapid exsanguination; resist the urge to explore any wounds that appear to breach platysma**
- **Ensure early senior medical attendance, direction, supervision and adequate imaging**

Examine for signs of:

- Airway injury
  — stridor, hoarse voice, haemoptysis, subcutaneous emphysema, anterior cartilaginous crepitus and/or tenderness

- Tension pneumothorax
  — tracheal deviation, distended neck veins
- Vascular injury
  — absent pulse, pulsatile haematoma, bruit, bleeding laceration
  — localizing neurological signs in the distribution of the carotid artery
- Nerve injury
  — sympathetic trunk (Horner's syndrome, phrenic (diaphragmatic paralysis), brachial plexus (upper limb signs)
- Cervical spine injury
  — tenderness, crepitus, step deformity, neurological deficit

CHEST

After primary survey chest injuries have been addressed, there still lurk insidious killers: mechanism of injury, clinical signs and CXR are the tools of choice

- Cardiac tamponade
  — penetrating trauma, hypotension, distended neck veins, usually normal cardiothoracic ratio (CTR)
- Traumatic aortic injury
  — high speed deceleration
  — suspicious mediastinum on CXR
  — pleural effusion
- Diaphragmatic hernia
  — abdominal compression injury
  — respiratory distress
  — poorly visualized diaphragm or bowel loops in hemithorax (left mostly)
- Oesophageal rupture
  — abdominal compression injury
  — mediastinal emphysema
  — pleural effusion
- Pneumothorax
  — suspect if subcutaneous emphysema
  — may be subclinical and not present on initial supine CXR
  — may only be evident after positive pressure ventilation
- Haemothorax
  — may be subtle and not present on initial supine CXR
  — Minor increases in hemithorax opacity may hide large blood volumes

- Myocardial contusion
  — associated with high speed and/or significant compressive force thoracic injury
  — precordial thoracic flail segments or sternal fractures with inner table involvement often associated
  — non-specific signs include tachycardia, hypotension in normovolaemic patient; an abnormal ECG is non-specific
  — cardiac enzyme levels correlate poorly with degree of injury
  — echocardiogram is the best diagnostic test

  Examine also for

- Contusions, lacerations, entrance/exit wounds
- Sternal fracture is common with airbag/seatbelt injury
- Rib fractures present with focal tenderness and crepitus. Sternal pressure with ribcage 'springing' helps to localize pain to areas suspicious for fracture. Subcutaneous emphysema suggests associated pneumothorax

> Cardiac tamponade is a penetrating injury phenomena;
> **it is extremely rare in blunt trauma**

ABDOMEN

After sources of major acute blood loss have been addressed or excluded in the primary survey, be wary of the following

A clear chest x-ray and normal pelvic x-ray in a haemodynamically unstable patient suggests the abdomen as the source for blood loss and the need for urgent laparotomy

- Traumatic bowel perforation
  — compressive abdominal injuries
  — 'seat belt' sign
  — abdominal tenderness
  — peritonism
  — 'free air' often absent on radiological studies
- Traumatic pancreatitis
  — direct abdominal trauma
  — 'handlebar' injury

> Bowel and mesenteric injuries are often not clinically evident in the acute phase even with 'negative CT abdomen' exams: admit and serially examine high-risk patients

- — fall from height
- — epigastric tenderness
- — raised lipase
- — CT and amylase are often insensitive and non-specific, respectively in the acute phase
- Renal injury
  - — consider in high speed motor vehicle collisions (MVC) or falls from significant height
  - — whilst contusions in the loin, lower ribs, renal angle suggest possible renal injury, absence does not exclude it
  - — absence of macroscopic or microscopic haematuria does *not* exclude renal injury and the degree of haematuria correlates poorly with degree of renal injury

PELVIS

- Pelvic palpation for pain/tenderness to detect pelvic disruption should be performed *once*, usually during the primary survey
- Repetitive stressing of pelvic fractures, including during log rolls and catheterization, increases bleeding by loss of initial haemostatic plugs and ongoing consumption of coagulation factors

> - Pelvic 'springing' should not be done
> - The sensitivity of pelvic springing is only 5% and is painful in the conscious patient

SPINE

After assessing the cervical spine, aim for a single logroll to assess for spinal injury.

- Enquire about subjective neck and back pain and assess distal neurostatus before logroll
- Make note of motor power, reflexes and sensory levels as part of the assessment for spinal injury

- Cervical spine best assessed with patient supine, collar released and in-line immobilization
- Thoracolumbar spine best examined at the time of logroll
- Palpate for tenderness, crepitus and step deformity
  — if negative, percuss the thoracolumbar spine to elicit areas of discomfort suggesting possible anterior structure injury (e.g. vertebral body wedge)
- Rectal examination for anal tone and/or sacral sparing (highly prognostic if present) should be performed at this stage
- Priapism as an autonomic reflex is not affected by neuromuscular blockade. Its presence may suggest spinal cord injury

> Interpreting neurological signs in the intubated, paralysed patient is very difficult.

- **Beware the occult spinal injury with penetrating gunshot wounds**
- **Up to 60% of bullets from non-exiting truncal gunshot wounds will be lodged in the spine**

PERINEUM

Perineal and rectal assessment should occur at the time of logroll.
  Look for signs of

- Urethral injury
  — blood at meatus of urethra
  — scrotal haematoma
  — high riding prostate on rectal examination
- Urethral injury is often present with significant pubic ramus, pelvic ring ('open book') or pelvic vertical disruption injuries

> - In males with any suspicion of urethral injury, a urethrogram should be performed prior to catheterization
> - This procedure is simple and can be performed in the resuscitation bay

Penetrating injuries of the buttocks and perineum should be regarded as intra-abdominal, intrapelvic or retroperitoneal until proven otherwise

- Vulval and vaginal injury
  — lacerations
  — per vaginal bleeding
- Rectal injury
  — lacerations
  — per rectal bleeding
  — rectal examination should determine the presence of anal tone, prostate position and the presence of blood or evidence of compound pelvic fractures

EXTREMITIES

Each limb should be examined for contusion, laceration, deformity, tenderness, crepitus and distal neurovascular status. With reference to positive findings from this initial assessment, functional active and passive range of movement should be tested, and each joint examined for effusion, tenderness, crepitus and ligamentous stability.

- Pedestrians involved in motor vehicle accidents not uncommonly have significant knee collateral ligament, menisci and tibial plateau injuries with relatively normal supine knee exams
- Be thorough and remember the mechanism of injury

- Compartment syndrome may occur in conjunction with crush injuries or fractures
  — severe neuropathic or ischaemic pain should raise suspicion
  — sensory dysfunction is usually the earliest sign; don't wait for absent pulses
  — compartment pressures should be measured to confirm

TERTIARY SURVEY

Background

The tertiary survey is a comprehensive review of the medical record of a major trauma patient combined with collation and review of all investigations and a complete head-to-toe examination.

Who does it?

- It is usually performed by the registrar of the admitting team within 24 h of the patient's admission
- Any clinician experienced in the assessment of major trauma may be suitable
- The findings are documented on a check sheet; further investigations, communications or treatment are then actioned immediately
- The tertiary survey should be repeated by the same clinician on weaning sedation or recovery of cognitive function, or if there is any new sign or symptom suggesting a missed injury

Why do it?

- The incidence of missed injuries following primary and secondary surveys is variable, but may be as high as 50% depending on how they are defined
- Missed injuries may lead to short- and long-term functional deficits, embarrassment of clinicians and litigation
- Formal tertiary surveys have been shown to reduce these rates by about 35%
- The remaining injuries are usually picked up within the following 2 weeks
- The commonest missed injuries are extremity fractures
- The patients at highest risk of missed injuries are those with severe brain injury, alcohol intoxication and those undergoing emergency surgery, all situations that may preclude a meaningful secondary survey
- To view an example of a tertiary survey form visit http://www.trauma.org/nurse/TertiaryTraumaSurvey.pdf

IMAGING TRIAGE IN MAJOR TRAUMA

Background

Physical examination and patient physiology are the cornerstones of clinical decision-making in trauma. Imaging techniques are now central to the accurate diagnosis and efficient treatment of most injured patients. CT, ultrasound (US) and interventional radiology (IR) have revolutionized trauma care. These modalities have increased the efficiency of diagnosis and significantly reduced the morbidity associated with unnecessary invasive diagnostic procedures and non-therapeutic/exploratory operations.

Assessment of severely injured patients has evolved into not only accurate 'injury identification' but also efficient 'injury exclusion'

The trauma team must be familiar with the appropriate use and interpretation of these radiological techniques to triage patients efficiently to operative intervention, monitoring on the ward, critical care or early discharge from the emergency department.

General principles of trauma imaging
The decision to use imaging, and the timing and choice of modality is guided by three factors.

- Patient physiology sets priorities
  — haemodynamic status
  — response to treatment
  — determines the risk of imaging: moving from the 'safety' of the resuscitation area to the 'risk' of the imaging suite
- Physical findings guide imaging needs
  — identifies anatomical region injured
  — based on specific signs and symptoms
- Mechanism of injury identifies the energy transfer sustained by the patient
  — penetrating mechanism: trajectory determination may help to define likely injuries
  — blunt mechanism: greater potential for multisystem energy transfer
  — requires a higher index of suspicion for multiregion injury

Considerations for the trauma team while making an imaging plan
- Are there obvious indications for immediate surgery?
  — should imaging be delayed until after surgical intervention?
- How will the imaging information alter/affect/improve the care of this patient?

A study that will not alter treatment, irrespective of its results, should not be done

- What is the risk of the procedure
  — intrinsic risk of the study itself (i.e. contrast, radiation, vascular access)

— risk of transport away from the resuscitation area
who will accompany the patient during the transfer?
what equipment will they need?
— risk of delaying treatments while continuing with diagnostic
testing
— remember that imaging is diagnostic *not* therapeutic
— what are the competing priorities between imaging and
therapeutic procedures?
• What is the risk of missing an injury if imaging is not
accomplished?

Initial evaluation

Imaging during the initial evaluation searches for bleeding and
treatable life-threatening conditions.

ATLS™ guidelines recommend the following:

1. Anteroposterior (AP) CXR: this must be the first imaging test
   performed irrespective of mechanism of injury or areas grossly
   injured
   • No patient should be transported out of the relative safety of
     the trauma resuscitation without the chest radiograph being
     reviewed by the trauma team
   • The physiological consequences of a missed pneumothorax
     (hypoxia and hypotension) far outweigh the benefits gained
     by having a head CT a few minutes earlier
2. AP pelvic film
   • Useful to identify major pelvic disruption or hip dislocation
     prior to leaving the resuscitation area
   • Recently considered to be optional in haemodynamically
     normal, asymptomatic patients who will undergo
     abdominopelvic CT during the secondary survey
   • Absolutely indicated in the following
     — haemodynamically unstable patients to search for pelvic
       source of bleeding
     — patients with physical findings consistent with hip
       dislocation or proximal femoral fracture requiring
       immediate reduction/stabilization
     — patients who will forego immediate CT in the event of
       emergent procedures
3. Cervical spine
   • Traditionally a three-view series: AP, lateral and odontoid
     view
   • Currently the literature is strongly in favour of omitting this
     series during the initial evaluation and including complete
     cervical spine CT in the secondary survey

HAEMODYNAMIC STATUS— IMAGING CONSIDERATIONS

The unstable patient

Imaging is done solely for the purpose of *cavitary triage*.

- Evaluate the chest, pericardium and abdomen/pelvis for life-threatening conditions or massive bleeding
- Quick, portable modalities are useful and the findings will not be subtle
  - portable (upright or reverse Trendelenburg if possible) chest radiograph to exclude massive haemothorax or tension pneumothorax
  - FAST examination to identify/exclude pericardial tamponade or massive intra-abdominal bleeding
  - pelvic plain film to identify major posterior element fracture: this may prompt the need for stabilization and/or embolization
- An unstable patient should *never* be taken to the CT scanner for *any* reason
- The interventional radiology suite is the only area in the radiology department where an unstable patient can get both diagnosis and treatment (haemorrhage control)

The stable patient

Imaging is an extension of the secondary survey to search and identify, or reliably exclude, injuries.

- Injury exclusion allows the clinician to triage resources (e.g. trauma bay beds, hospital beds, ICU beds), reserving them for more injured patients
- Specific imaging algorithms are based on mechanism of injury, index of suspicion and physical findings

PENETRATING TRAUMA

After penetrating trauma, imaging is used to help identify trajectory.

> Trajectory determination equals injury identification

- Radio-opaque markers should be placed on all penetrating wounds to 'see' the trajectory between the otherwise invisible soft tissue defects

- Paper clips opened into a triangle and taped onto the patient so that the wound is in the centre of the triangle are ideal bullet markers

> Radio-opaque markers should be placed on all penetrating wounds

Craniofacial
- CT is the only study for penetrating trauma to the cranium and typically serves prognostic purposes only
- Plain radiographs serve no clinical purpose in this setting
- There is rarely an indication for repeat studies, irrespective of clinical course
- Angiography is recommended if vascular injury is suspected
- Magnetic resonance imaging (MRI) is not recommended (the reason being that bullets/fragments may be moved by the magnetic field)

Neck
- The anatomical complexity of the neck requires the evaluation and triage of three groups of structures irrespective of the level or zone of penetration
  — pharynx/oesophagus
  — airway/trachea
  — cerebral vessels
- Imaging after penetrating neck trauma has undergone a revolution in the recent past. Two approaches are described: the traditional and the modern

Traditional
Penetrations are grouped by zone of injury (Fig. 1.9).

- Zone 1: panendoscopy, barium swallow, four-vessel angiogram
- Zone 2: mandatory exploration of all structures (or panendoscopy, barium swallow, four-vessel angiogram)
- Zone 3: panendoscopy, barium swallow, four-vessel angiogram

Modern
Irrespective of zone of injury.

- Haemodynamically normal patients without hard signs of vascular or aerodigestive injury
  — CT angiogram to identify missile trajectory and to triage 'at-risk' structures based on the path of penetration

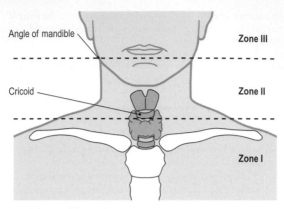

Figure 1.9 Zones of the neck

- Follow-up testing with endoscopy, barium radiographs, or selective angiography is performed to evaluate at-risk structures

Chest
- All patients require a CXR—upright if possible—to identify haemothorax/pneumothorax and trajectory
- Ultrasound pericardial view (FAST examination) approaches 100% sensitivity for cardiac injury
- Transmediastinal trajectories require the evaluation of the digestive tract, heart and great vessels, and the tracheobronchial tree
  — similar to neck penetration, evaluation of stable patients with injuries that traverse the mediastinum
  traditional: chest radiograph followed by angiography, bronchoscopy, oesophagoscopy, oesophagography and pericardial window
  modern: directed approach—chest radiograph, pericardial ultrasound triage, CT angiography with subsequent treatment or directed radiographic/endoscopic evaluation of structures 'at risk for injury based on trajectory

Abdomen/retroperitoneum
- Unstable patients with abdominal penetration are candidates for cavitary triage with portable chest radiograph and FAST
- FAST is highly sensitive in unstable patients to identify the bleeding cavity (Fig. 1.10)

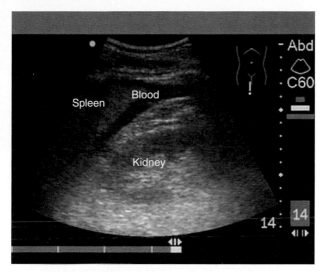

Figure 1.10 Focused assessment with sonography for trauma (FAST)

- Plain films with penetrating wounds marked by radio-opaque markers are used to identify trajectory
- Complete torso imaging (chest, abdomen and pelvis) should occur with all thoracoabdominal penetrating wounds
- Haemodynamically normal patients with back, flank or tangential-appearing penetrations are candidates for selective management based on physical examination and imaging findings
    — FAST
      a positive FAST in this setting precludes the need for further imaging
      sensitivity is only 46–67% in stable penetrating trauma patients, therefore a negative study *requires* further evaluation
    — contrast-enhanced abdominal CT can identify trajectory and is sensitive (near 100%) for gunshot wounds, peritoneal penetration or retroperitoneal injury
      abdominal CT may not accurately diagnose diaphragmatic injuries

Extremity
- Plain radiographs will accurately diagnose long bone fractures and will identify trajectory

- Angiography may be needed to assess the vasculature in selected patients without hard signs of vascular injury (see p. 175 Peripheral vascular injury)
  — angiography should not delay surgery if hard signs of vascular injury are present
  — often an 'on-table' angiogram is appropriate to identify the level of injury if multiple penetrations exist
  — completion 'on-table' angiography is highly recommended after vascular repair

BLUNT TRAUMA

Craniofacial

- CT is the imaging modality of choice to identify/exclude traumatic brain injury after blunt trauma
  — all patients with depressed mental status, loss of consciousness, amnesia or evidence of direct cranial trauma should undergo non-contrast CT
  — the negative predictive value of a normal head CT in a patient with mild traumatic brain injury (loss of consciousness/amnesia) is 99.7%, indicating that such patients can safely be discharged with family/friends if further work-up is negative
  — repeat scanning within 24 h to evaluate progression is common after an abnormal initial head CT
    the clinical value of this is not supported by evidence if there is no change in clinical status/physical examination
- Clinical suspicion of facial fractures should prompt the emergency team to obtain fine-cut imaging data through the mandible at the time of initial CT with three-dimensional reconstructions to avoid repeating studies

Neck

- Radiographic evaluation of the cervical spine is indicated in all patients who cannot be reliably examined clinically owing to altered mental status, neck pain or distracting injury
  — three-view plain film cervical spine radiographs appear to be inadequate to reliably exclude injury in a large proportion of patients after blunt trauma
  — complete cervical spine CT with coronal and sagittal reconstructions are sensitive and specific for cervical spine fractures

— ligamentous injury can be identified on flexion–extension views in alert patients, but is more reliably diagnosed in both alert and comatose patients with MRI
— blunt cerebrovascular injury
aggressive screening has increased the awareness of this uncommon entity. The following injuries warrant screening:
  a. mechanism of severe hyperextension/rotation – LeFort II/III facial fractures
  b. diffuse axonal injury of the brain
  c. near-hanging
  d. seatbelt abrasion of anterior neck
  e. basilar skull fracture involving the carotid canal
  f. cervical vertebral body fracture
CT angiogram and MRI/magnetic resonance angiography (MRA) have been studied as screening modalities. Prospective data indicate sensitivities/specificities less than 70% each
four-vessel angiography remains the gold standard for diagnosis
risks of angiogram must be weighed against the index of suspicion and the willingness to accept the insensitive nature of computed tomographic angiography (CTA) and MRI/MRA

Spine
- Imaging of the complete thoracic and/or lumbar spines is indicated in any patient who has tenderness on physical examination, neurological symptoms consistent with spinal injury, or impaired mental status preventing adequate physical examination
  — plain films: AP and lateral radiographs are often technically inadequate owing to body habitus: sensitivity <60%; specificity 93%. Further, portable machines cannot image the entire spine, necessitating transport to the radiology department
  — axial CT combined with AP/lateral CT scanograms are adequate to screen for lumbar spinal fractures
  — axial CT with three-dimensional reconstructions of the thoracolumbar spine is highly sensitive and specific (97% and 99%, respectively) and requires no additional time or radiation exposure after CT of the chest/abdomen/pelvis

Chest

- Plain AP chest radiographs are critical to rule out life-threatening conditions such as pneumothorax and haemothorax
- Blunt aortic disruption: although neither sensitive nor specific, certain CXR findings suggest further evaluation
  — widened mediastinum (>8 cm)
  — obliteration of aortic knob
  — obliteration of aortopulmonary window
  — deviation of trachea to right
  — presence of pleural cap
  — depression of the left mainstem bronchus >40°
  — deviation of oesophagus (nasogastric tube) to right
- Angiography is the gold standard for the diagnosis of aortic disruption after blunt trauma
- Chest CT is more commonly used to evaluate thoracic trauma
  — detect occult pneumothoraces
  — diagnose and characterize sternal, scapular and multiple rib fractures
  — triage the mediastinal structures for vascular disruption in cases of abnormal CXR findings or in cases of significant deceleration. Although a sensitive screening tool, the poor specificity of chest CT for aortic disruption usually requires angiographic confirmation prior to surgery
  — diagnosis of pulmonary contusion

Abdomen/retroperitoneum

Abdominal CT has become the most widely used tool for evaluating the abdomen after blunt trauma. This modality has been heavily studied with the following conclusions.

Abdominal CT

Abdominal CT is useful in evaluating the following:

- Assess and grade solid organ injuries: useful for prognosis and management decisions
  — contrast blush is useful in determining the need for angiographic embolization
  diagnose and characterize pelvic fractures
  diagnose and characterize lumbar spine and sacral fractures
  assess retroperitoneal structures for injury
  diagnose most cases of hollow viscus injury
  — CT has a false-negative rate of 10–13% for hollow viscus injury

— CT findings consistent with hollow viscus injury are:
  1. Hard signs: free air and oral contrast extravasation
  2. Soft signs: free fluid, bowel thickening, mesenteric 'stranding' and haematoma
— selective repeats of abdominal CT may increase the sensitivity in diagnosing hollow viscus injury
- The negative predictive value of a 'normal' contrast-enhanced abdominal CT is 99.63% irrespective of physical examination findings
- The routine use of oral contrast is not supported by prospective data
- Routine repeat abdominal CT to assess solid organs after non-operative management is not needed

Focused assessment with sonography for trauma (FAST)
- Three-view assessment of the right upper quadrant, left upper quadrant and pelvis
- Limited sensitivity (86%) in assessing routine blunt abdominal trauma in stable patients
  — negative exams require a follow-up modality (serial physical examinations, serial ultrasounds or abdominal CT) to exclude injury
- Highly sensitive (100%) for blunt abdominal injury in cases of haemodynamic instability
- Plain abdominal radiographs have no role in assessing blunt abdominal trauma
- Angiography is useful to control bleeding from solid organs or pelvic fractures. Contrast blush on abdominal CT typically prompts angiographic evaluation for active bleeding

Extremity
- Plain radiographs are the standard for the diagnosis and characterization of extremity fractures due to blunt trauma
- Increasingly, extremity CT is being used by orthopaedic surgeons to more fully characterize complex fractures after plain film evaluation
- MRI is useful to assess ligamentous and soft tissue injury
- Angiography is indicated to evaluate the peripheral vasculature after fractures or dislocations if there are signs of vascular injury on physical examination

SYSTEMS

HEAD AND NECK

TRAUMATIC BRAIN INJURY

Background
Survival and overall outcome from traumatic brain injury are dependent on rapid identification of the injury and immediate initiation of treatment to prevent secondary brain injury.

> Traumatic brain injury is a leading cause of mortality in trauma

> Loss of consciousness (LOC) – whether brief or prolonged LOC is a predictor of traumatic brain injury

Identification
- Glasgow Coma Scale (GCS; Table 2.1)
  — standardized objective assessment of the severity of head injury
  — numerical scores are assigned to the *best* motor, verbal and eye-opening response
  — the highest score obtained is 15, signifying a neurologically normal patient
  — the minimal score is 3, seen in moribund/comatose patients
  — a good motor response is the best early predictor of outcome
- Pupillary response
  — evaluates the second and third cranial nerves and midbrain
  — unilateral reactive dilated pupil suggests mass effect of the temporal lobe or an epidural haematoma in the middle fossa
- Hemiparesis/hemiplegia
  — arises from mass-occupying lesions on the side opposite the neurological deficit
- Cheyne–Stokes respirations
  — cycles of hyperventilation followed by apnoea
  — seen in severe traumatic brain injury with impending herniation

Head CT scan is the radiographic gold standard for the identification of TBI
   Rapidly performed in stabilized patients with abnormal neurological exam and/or LOC

TABLE 2.1 Glasgow Coma Scale

Eye opening	Score	Verbal response	Score	Motor response	Score
Spontaneous	4	Oriented	5	Follows commands	6
To command	3	Confused	4	Localizes to pain	5
To pain	2	Verbalizes	3	Withdraws to pain	4
None	1	Vocalizes	2	Flexion (decorticate)	3
		None	1	Extension (decerebrate)	2
				None	1

*Intubated patients are signified with a 't', i.e. intubated comatose = 3t

Types of brain injury

- Concussion
  - transient loss of consciousness, no findings on computed tomography (CT) scan
  - repetitive concussions may have longlasting neuropsychological effects
- Epidural/extradural haematoma
  - *neurosurgical emergency if mass effect*
  - arterial bleeding, usually middle meningeal artery, between skull and dura mater
  - 'lucid interval' of consciousness before rapid central nervous system (CNS) deterioration
- Subdural haematoma
  - *neurosurgical emergency if mass effect*
  - most common (20–40%), usually venous bleeding, slow deterioration
  - arises from bleeding small veins bridging between dura mater and arachnoid membrane
- Subarachnoid haemorrhage
  - diffuse layering of blood below arachnoid membrane
  - does not cause mass effect, predisposes to vasospasm
- Cerebral contusion
  - *neurosurgical emergency if mass effect*
  - intracerebral haematomas occur from direct parenchymal injury
  - may progress in size due to continued bleeding (24 h) or oedema (72 h)
- Diffuse axonal injury
  - loss of gray–white matter interface on CT scan, better shown on magnetic resonance imaging (MRI)
  - axonal disruption due to cerebral shear forces

Severity of brain injury

Traumatic brain injury may be characterized using the GCS into minor, moderate and severe (Table 2.2).

TABLE 2.2 Severity of head injury	
Severity	*GCS*
Minor	14–15
Moderate	9–13
Severe	<9

Minor brain injury
- Mild confusion without loss of consciousness (LOC) or brief LOC at time of injury
- GCS 14–15
- Head CT scan without abnormality
- Mortality <1%
- No impairments
  GCS score 14 and 15 warrant admission if:
- CT scan is negative but patient presents with severe physiological manifestations of a concussion, including:
  — loss of consciousness
  — headache
  — nausea and vomiting
  — diplopia
  — short-term memory loss or perseveration
  — *in other words if there are patient safety issues that require close supervision*
- CT scan of the brain shows intracranial or extracranial blood, i.e. contusion, subarachnoid or subdural haemorrhage, etc.
  — there is growing evidence that small subarachnoid haemorrhages or small amounts of extra-axial blood require neither antiseizure prophylaxis nor repeat CT scan
  — the use of seizure prophylaxis in these patients remains contentious and national guidelines differ in their recommendations: confirm local policies
    although some centres continue to recommend repeat CT scan in this group its diagnostic value is really limited to patients who have had a change in GCS

Moderate brain injury
- GCS score 9–13
- Neurosurgical deterioration occurs in 10%
- LOC >5 min or continued confusion at time of assessment
- Head CT scan with non-surgical abnormality
- Mortality <3%
- May have physical, cognitive, behavioural impairments

Patients with moderate brain injury:

- Require repeated examination in 1–2 h
  — all patients with a GCS of 9–13 are admitted to an intensive care unit (ICU) or high dependency unit (HDU)
- Absolute need for repeated CT scan within 24 h or sooner if:
  — decrease in GCS by two or more points
    motor score most predictive
    check for narcotic or sedative administration

- Intracranial pressure (ICP) monitoring may be warranted in moderate brain injury if the patient is going to the operating room for a long procedure

- Patients who deteriorate to GCS of 9 or less must have their airway controlled, especially if moving to CT scan or the theatre
- These patients cannot protect their airway and are vulnerable to even one episode of hypoxaemia

Severe brain injury
- GCS ≤8
- Altered level of consciousness/neurological impairment at time of assessment
- All patients require admission to ICU and active therapy to control blood pressure and ICP as needed
- Elevated ICP
- Head CT scan with abnormality may require surgical intervention
- Mortality >20%
- Significant physical, cognitive, behavioural impairments likely
- These patients are vulnerable to secondary brain injury from hypoxia (saturation <90%, hypotension: mean arterial pressure <80 mmHg, cerebral perfusion pressure <60 mmHg)
- Other secondary insults include hyperglycaemia, hyperthermia and anaemia

- Hypotension alone increases mortality in severe traumatic brain injury from 27% to 60%
- Hypoxia with hypotension increases mortality to 75%

Initial treatment

Stabilization and prevention of secondary injury
- <C> Catastrophic haemorrhage
  — address and control sources of catastrophic haemorrhage
- Airway
  — supplemental O_2 to maintain saturation >94%
  — if GCS ≤8, rapid sequence intubation
  — use short-acting medications, allowing frequent neurological examinations

- Breathing
  — address life-threatening injuries
  — support ventilation as required
  — prevent any hypoxia
  — do not hyperventilate
- Circulation support
  — obtain venous access
  — resuscitation with isotonic fluids (normal saline) or blood
  — maintain mean arterial pressure ≥90 mmHg
- Disability
  — obtain baseline initial neurological exam
    best if performed prior to administration of paralytics for
      intubation
  — reduce intracranial pressure
    reverse Trendelenburg position
    mannitol 0.5–1.0 g/kg i.v. if rapid CNS deterioration or signs
      of lateralization
    do not hyperventilate: maintain $PaCO_2$ at 35 mmHg
  — rapidly obtain head CT
    if physiologically stable, head CT prior to operative
      intervention for other injuries will enable neurosurgical
      treatment during any operative treatment
  — maintain spine immobilization
    8% of patients with traumatic brain injury have a cervical
      spine injury
  — obtain laboratory tests
    prothrombin time (PT), partial thromboplastin time (PTT),
      international normalized ratio (INR), fibrinogen: fresh
      frozen plasma (FFP) and cryoprecipitate as indicated
    full blood count (FBC): maintain haematocrit of 30% to
      maximize oxygen-carrying capacity
    arterial blood gases: PaO_2 >70 mmHg and $PaCO_2$ of
      30–35 mmHg

*Early neurosurgical intervention is required if GCS ≤8, mass effect
seen on CT scan.*

Frequently asked questions

1. Which patients require antiseizure therapy?
   - Generally speaking, if a seizure occurs during the acute
     traumatic event no treatment is necessary
   - The need for *seizure prophylaxis* is dependent on the amount
     of intracranial or extra-axial haemorrhage and is usually
     continued for 7 days

- If a seizure occurs at any time *after* the initial event, therapy should be started as per local protocol
- Intensivist and neurosurgeon should decide treatment courses together
- If a patient with traumatic brain injury with a GCS of 3 is intubated, it is very difficult to observe seizure activity, and seizure prophylaxis should be considered in these patients as well

2. What role do steroids have in patients with traumatic brain injury?
   - Currently there is no proven benefit from steroid use in traumatic brain injury

3. When should hyperventilation be used?
   - It is now well established that hyperventilation worsens overall cerebral ischaemia, and the penumbra or zone of injury adjacent to directly traumatized brain is most at risk
   - There is no longer an indication for routine hyperventilation of patients to a PCO_2 of 25 mmHg (3.5 kPa) except in suspected impending brain herniation. This will sustain the patient either to CT scan or to the operating theatre

SPINE INJURY

CERVICAL SPINE

Background

- The incidence of cervical spine injuries is 1–3% among blunt trauma survivors
- The incidence of missed C-spine injuries is reported to be between 5 and 30%
- The most commonly missed injuries are C1–C2 and C7–T1
- The appropriate method of evaluating the C-spine is widely debated in the literature
- Less than one-third of patients with a spinal fracture have a neurological deficit

Basics of cervical spine precautions

- All blunt trauma patients should be placed in spinal precautions until examination is complete

 Assume all blunt trauma patients have a cervical spine injury until proven otherwise!

- Penetrating trauma to the neck has a low incidence of unstable C-spine injuries
- A hard C-collar should be placed on all blunt trauma patients
  — the type of hard collar is less important than ensuring a proper fit
- Hard collars do not immobilize the neck completely
  — if an incomplete C-spine injury is suspected, taping the head to the backboard, or additional manual stabilization with sandbags, is advisable
- The C-collar should never interfere with a complete clinical examination of the neck
  — manual in-line stabilization should be held while the collar is removed for examination or intubation

Who does *not* need radiographic evaluation of the cervical spine?

This has been the subject of some debate and a number of studies. Currently the Canadian C-spine rule is preferred.

- ATLS™, 1997
  — no films needed 'for patients who are awake, alert, sober, and neurologically normal, and have no neck pain'
- East (2000 update): Level II recommendation
  — cervical spine films are not necessary for patients who are 'alert, awake, not intoxicated, neurologically normal, no midline neck pain or tenderness even with full range of motion of neck and palpation of cervical spine'
- NEXUS: National Emergency X-Radiography Utilization Study (Hoffman et al 2000, 2002)
  — patients must meet all five criteria
  no midline cervical tenderness
  no focal neurological deficit
  normal alertness
  no intoxication
  no painful, distracting injury
- CCR: Canadian C-Spine Rule for Radiography in Alert and Stable Trauma Patients (Stiell et al 2001)

  Three-step pathway in patients who are alert (GCS 15) and stable:

1. Any high-risk factors?
   - If any 'yes' then x-rays
   - Age ≥65 years

- Dangerous mechanism
  — fall from elevation ≥3 feet or five stairs
  — an axial load to head (e.g. diving)
  — a motor vehicle collision at high speed (>100 km/h) or with rollover or ejection
  — a collision involving a motorized recreational vehicle
  — a bicycle collision
- Paraesthesias in extremities

2. Any low-risk factor that allows safe assessment of range of motion?
   - If 'no' then take films
   - Simple rear end motor vehicle collision
   - Sitting position in emergency department
   - Ambulatory at any time
   - Delayed onset of neck pain
   - Absence of midline C-spine tenderness

3. Able to rotate neck actively 45° left and right?
   - If 'no' then take films

CCR is superior to NEXUS low-risk criteria with respect to sensitivity and specificity for C-spine injury (Stiell et al 2003).

What is the appropriate radiographic study? (See Chapter 1 Imaging)

Cervical spine radiographs
- 3-view: anteroposterior (AP), lateral and odontoid

If the above criteria are fulfilled, no radiographic studies are needed, the C-spine can be cleared clinically, and the collar removed

---

Canadian C-spine rule
Blunt trauma spines can be cleared clinically if:
1. There are no distracting injuries
2. GCS = 15
3. No cervical, thoracic, lumbar tenderness
4. No neurological impairments
5. Normal physiology
6. Patient able to rotate neck 45°
7. Low force mechanism

Clinical clearance of the cervical spine
The clinical examination requires an alert,
non-intoxicated patient that can focus on the doctor and
the neck exam without distraction.
- Ask the patient if they have any neck pain. *If 'no',
proceed*
- Perform a gross motor and sensory exam. *If 'normal',
proceed*
- Remove the C-collar and stabilize the neck with gentle
pressure on the forehead of the patient. Palpate each
vertebra and ask the patient whether pain is elicited
during palpation. *If 'no', proceed*
- Apply vertical pressure on the patient's skull and ask
the patient about pain. *If 'no', proceed*
- Ask the patient to move their head forward ('chin to
chest'), back ('chin to ceiling'), and laterally ('chin to
shoulder'). Ask if there is any pain during movement. *If
'no', remove collar*
- If pain is elicited during any of the above manoeuvres,
replace the C-collar and proceed with radiographic
evaluation

- 5-view: AP, lateral, odontoid and obliques
  — adequate films must visualize the entire C-spine (C1 to the
  top of T1)
  — additional swimmers' view may be required
  — plain films alone may miss 45–55% of injuries
- Flexion/extension: lateral of C1–T1 while patient is flexing and
  extending the neck *actively*
  — patient must be awake, alert and cooperative
  — inadequate if <30° of flexion and extension
  — motion must be voluntary and painless
  — identifies motion as a result of ligamentous instability

Cervical spine CT
- This is increasingly the preferred modality
- Axial images with sagittal and coronal reconstructions
- Useful to image C1–C2 and C6–T1 and any tender or abnormal
  area on plain films
- May be obtained of entire cervical spine, in place of plain films,
  if obtaining CT images of other body regions
- Does not evaluate for ligamentous injury

Cervical spine MRI
- Evaluates for ligamentous injury and spinal cord abnormalities

> If radiographs are ordered, a minimum of three views is
> required and must be adequate to evaluate C1–T1

Systematic review of cervical spine radiographs

Lateral radiograph
- Should include skull base to top of T1
- Inspect alignment of posterior vertebral line, anterior vertebral line and spinolaminar line (Fig. 2.1)
- Soft-tissue space
    — no greater than 5 mm at C2 vertebral body
    — no greater than 20 mm at C6 vertebral body
    — atlantodens interval: the space between the anterior aspect of the odontoid and the ring of C1
       no greater than 3.5 mm in adult
       no greater than 5 mm in a child
- Vertebral height should be symmetrical anterior and posterior
- Loss of normal cervical lordosis (straightening of the spine) indicates extensor muscle spasm and can suggest spinal injury

Open-mouth odontoid
- Dens should be fully visualized and should be symmetrically located between the lateral masses of C1
- Lateral masses of C1 in relationship to C2
    — little or no overhang of the lateral masses should be seen
    — overhang of >6.5 mm indicates fracture of the ring of C1

Figure 2.2 shows normal open-mouth odontoid views.

Anteroposterior radiograph
- Distance between spinous processes
- Alignment
- Rotation

  **Cervical fractures have a 16–20% incidence of a distal
non-contiguous spinal fracture. Imaging of the entire
axial spine is recommended**

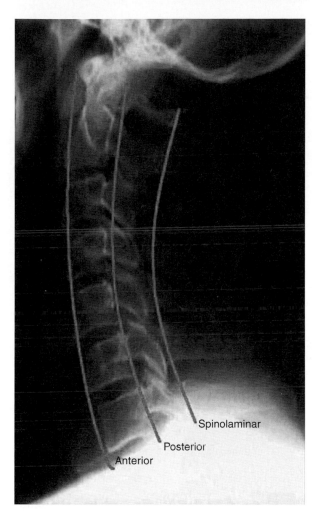

Figure 2.1 Normal lateral radiograph with demonstration of the anterior vertebral body line, posterior vertebral body line and spinolaminar line

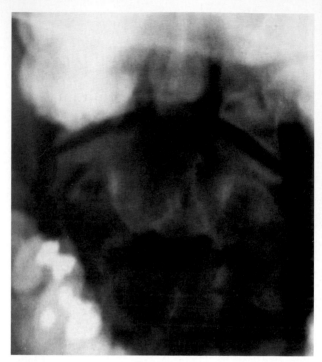

Figure 2.2 Normal open-mouth odontoid images

THORACIC AND LUMBAR SPINE

Background

- 50–70% of thoracolumbar spine injuries occur between T10 and L2
- Mechanisms include motor vehicle collisions (40%), violence (36%), sports (15%) and falls (7.5%)
- 70% of thoracolumbar injuries will have *no* neurological deficit at presentation

- **Patients should be removed from the spine board as soon as possible**
- **Spine precautions are maintained by logrolling the patient**

Clinical examination
- Roll the patient, maintaining axial spine alignment
- Inspect the spine for localized swelling or deformity
- Palpate the entire spinal column. Ask the patient if tenderness is present. Palpate for step-offs or widening between spinous processes
- Perform a thorough neurological examination, including rectal tone reflex

Radiographic evaluation
- Plain films
  — AP and lateral images of the thoracic and lumbar spine
  — AP to evaluate distance between pedicles and spinous processes, evaluate transverse processes and ribs for fractures
  — lateral to evaluate anterior and posterior lines and vertebral height
- CT
  — spiral CT with sagittal and coronal reconstructions further evaluates abnormalities seen on plain films diagnostic test of choice to delineate bony anatomy
- MRI
  — useful to evaluate integrity of spinal ligaments and spinal cord
  — indicated for all patients with neurological deficits

Column spinal support
- Anterior column: anterior longitudinal ligament and the anterior two-thirds of the vertebral body and disc
- Middle column: posterior third of the vertebral body and disc, and the posterior longitudinal ligament
- Posterior column: the facet joints, capsule, ligamentum flavum and posterior longitudinal ligaments

> Fractures or injuries of two of three columns denotes biomechanical instability and may require surgical stabilization. A spine specialist should be consulted

REFERENCES

Advanced trauma life support for doctors course manual, 6th edn 1997
American College of Surgeons, Chicago ATLS

Eastern Association for the Surgery of Trauma 1998 Practice management guidelines for identifying cervical spine injuries following trauma. EAST practice parameter workgroup for cervical spine clearance. http://www.east.org/tpg/chap3.pdf. Accessed online January 2007

Hoffman J R, Mower W R, Wolfson A B et al 2000 Validity of a set of clinical criteria to rule out injury to the cervical spine in patients with blunt trauma. National emergency X-radiography utilization study group. The New England Journal of Medicine 343(2):94–99 (Erratum in The New England Journal of Medicine 344(6):464)

Stiell I G, Wells G A, Vandemheen K L et al 2001 The Canadian C-spine rule for radiography in alert and stable trauma patients. The Journal of the American Medical Association 286(15):1841–1848

Stiell I G, Clement C M, McKnight R D et al 2003 The Canadian C-spine rule versus the NEXUS low-risk criteria in patients with trauma. The New England Journal of Medicine 349(26):2510–2518

FURTHER READING

Marion D W, Domeier R 1998 Practice management guidelines for identifying cervical spine instability after trauma. Journal of Trauma 44:945–946

SPINAL CORD INJURY

Background

- 50–60% of spinal cord injuries involve the cervical spine
- There is a bimodal distribution of injuries, with a peak in adolescents and young adults (15–30 years) and a second smaller peak around age 50–70 years due to degenerative disease
- A large number of cervical spine injuries with a neurological deficit may be immediately fatal secondary to cardiorespiratory compromise
- Neurogenic shock with hypotension and bradycardia is frequently encountered in patients with spinal cord injury above C5–C6, but can be seen with more distal injuries

Diagnosis

- The diagnosis of spinal cord injury is made on clinical grounds
- The level of spinal cord injury usually correlates with the level of spinal column injury
- Spinal cord injury can occur without spinal column injury
- The diagnosis of spinal cord injury is supplemented with MRI
- Radiographic evaluation using plain film or CT (see Spine Injury) is required to plan operative intervention

- MRI
  - identification of ligamentous spine injury, nerve root compression or cord injury
  - 0.05% incidence of pure ligamentous injury
  - 65% incidence of ligamentous injury with spine fracture
- Magnetic resonance angiography (MRA)/angiogram
  - Four-vessel imaging (vertebral and carotids)
  - 13–17% incidence of blunt vertebral artery injury with C-spine fractures

Neurological evaluation

- Mental status
  - GCS should be recorded
- Cranial nerve examination
  - pay special attention to third nerve and pupillary size and symmetry
- Motor examination
  - each extremity should be evaluated individually
  - strength is evaluated according to American Spinal Injury Assessment (ASIA) protocol (Table 2.3)
- Sensory testing
  - light touch and pinprick along dermatome levels
  - impairment of pain sensation and temperature may indicate central cord or Brown–Sequard syndrome
- Reflex testing
  - biceps, triceps, brachioradialis, knee and ankles
  - Babinski responses should be recorded as present or absent

> The neurological level of injury is determined and recorded as the most caudal segment of the spinal cord with normal sensory and motor function on both sides of the body

TABLE 2.3 Muscle strength grading system	
Grade	Findings
5	Normal strength
4	Overcomes moderate resistance
3	Full range of motion against gravity only
2	Full range of motion with gravity eliminated
1	Trace muscle contraction on palpation
0	Flaccid

ASIA impairment scale
- Used to grade impairment as complete or incomplete (Table 2.4)

Clinical syndromes
- Spinal cord concussion
  — 4% incidence
  — temporary loss of neurological function for 24–48 h
  — usually deceleration injury with pre-existing spinal stenosis
  — resolves with supportive treatment, no long-term disabilities
- Complete spinal cord injury
  — 42% incidence
  — loss of all motor and sensory function below level of pathology
  — results in quadriplegia or paraplegia based on level of injury
  — lifelong disability
- Incomplete spinal cord injury
  — 52% incidence
  — preservation of sensory or motor function below the level of injury
- Central cord syndrome
  — usually elderly patients with pre-existing spinal stenosis
  — cord contusion causes ischaemia to central portion of cord
  — motor and sensory deficits greater in the upper than in the lower extremities
  — bowel and bladder function is impaired
  — lower extremity nervous tracts are lateral whereas upper extremity tracts are central
  — 50% of patients will have long-term disability

TABLE 2.4 ASIA impairment scale	
A	Complete loss of sensory and motor function (including sacral area) below the level of neurological injury
B	Incomplete injury, where sensation is preserved below the level of neurological injury, including the sacral area
C	Incomplete injury with motor function preserved below the level of neurological injury and most preserved groups exhibiting strength of ≤3
D	Incomplete injury with motor function preserved below the level of neurological injury and most preserved groups exhibiting strength of ≥3
E	Normal sensory and motor examination

- Brown–Sequard syndrome
  — injury, usually penetrating, to lateral half of spinal cord
  — loss of ipsilateral motor and proprioception
  — loss of contralateral pain and temperature sensation
  — injury to lateral spinothalamic tracts below decussation of fibres
  — prognosis is poor, with permanent disabilities
- Anterior cord syndrome
  — injury is from ischaemia or trauma (bone fragments) to the anterior cord
  — loss of motor, pain and temperature sensation below level of injury
  — vibration and proprioception is preserved (dorsal cord)
  — prognosis poor, with <10% regaining motor function
- Conus medullaris syndrome
  — injury to the sacral cord (conus) and lumbar nerve roots within the spinal canal
  — results in areflexic bladder, bowel and lower limbs
  — sacral segments may show preserved reflexes (bulbocavernosus and micturition reflexes)
- Bilateral lower extremity motor and sensory deficits
  — bowel and bladder dysfunction occurs, minimal pain seen
  — early operative decompression is vital for long-term recovery
- Cauda equina syndrome
  — injury to the lumbosacral nerve roots within the neural canal
  — asymmetric radicular pain of lower extremities
  — results in areflexic bladder, bowel and lower limbs

Management

- <C> Catastrophic haemorrhage
  — address life-threatening haemorrhage
- Airway
  — casualties with a GCS <9 require intubation for airway protection
  — immobilize with hard cervical collar and in-line cervical stabilization
  — maintain logroll precautions
- Breathing
  — progressive respiratory compromise may result from high C-spine and thoracic spine injuries, and early intubation should be considered
- Circulation
  — hypotension should be treated promptly to avoid secondary cord injury
  — initial treatment should be fluid administration

> Hypotension should be regarded as a sign of haemorrhagic shock in the blunt trauma patient before considering neurogenic shock

Specific management
- Steroid (glucocorticoid) protocol
  — remains controversial
  — in a series of double-blinded studies (NASCIS I, II and III), the use of glucocorticoids has not been *conclusively* shown to have significant impact on spinal cord injuries
  — subgroup analysis of this data has suggested that patients with complete and incomplete injuries after non-penetrating trauma may have beneficial motor and sensory effects at 6 weeks, 6 months and 1 year.
  — local policies should be followed

Dosing of methylprednisolone (start only if <8 h from injury)
- Initial bolus 30 mg/kg i.v. over 45 min
- Start continuous infusion of 5.4 mg/kg/h i.v.
- Continue for 23 h if started <3 h from injury
- Continue for 48 h if started between 3–8 h from injury

- Complete radiographic evaluation
- Consult spine specialist
- Preventative measures
  — place nasogastric tube and Foley: paralytic ileus and bladder atony are common
  — heating and cooling blankets may be needed secondary to loss of thermoregulation
  — aggressive pulmonary toilet, rotating beds and tracheostomy may be needed for prevention of pulmonary complications
  — decubitus ulcer prevention is paramount in the insensate patient
  — stress gastric ulcer prophylaxis (especially with high-dose steroids)
  — thromboembolism prophylaxis
  — physical therapy may help prevent joint contractures and heterotopic ossification

- Dysautonomia
  - exaggerated sympathetic and parasympathetic responses to simple stimuli such as cough, gag or Valsalva manoeuvre
  - bradycardia is most common, and may require atropine or pacemaker placement
  - usually temporary, but can last from a few weeks to even a year
- Spinal shock
  - spinal shock should be differentiated from neurogenic shock
  - this is a neurological phenomenon, not haemodynamic
  - this is the spinal equivalent to a concussion of the brain
  - results in flaccidity, loss of distal segmental reflexes and loss of bulbocavernosus reflex
  - most patients recover within 5–10 days, but recovery may take several months

Neurogenic shock
- Seen in spinal cord injuries above T6
- Results from disruption of autonomic pathways maintaining cardiac output and peripheral vascular tone
- Characterized by hypotension, bradycardia and hypothermia
- ↓Cardiac output, ↓systemic vascular resistance, ↓pulmonary arterial wedge pressure, ↓central venous pressure
- Establish a normal central venous pressure with volume administration
- Augment blood pressure and heart rate with vasoconstrictors and chronotropic agents
  - dopamine, noradrenaline (norepinephrine), atropine, ephedrine

 Haemorrhagic shock must be ruled out in all cases of hypotension

Outcomes
- Spinal cord injuries are physically and psychologically devastating
- Up to 90% of patients with traumatic quadriplegia eventually return home with some form of functional independence
  - approximately 200 000 people live in the United States with a disability resulting from spinal cord injury
  - 32% of paraplegics and 25% of quadriplegics are able to return to employment after injury

- For patients who survive their initial hospitalization, average life expectancy can range from 1 to 4 decades (Table 2.5)
- Recurrent hospitalizations, especially in the elderly, are frequently required to treat the associated complications of immobility
- Life expectancy is better in incomplete injury, paraplegia, young age at time of injury and low quadriplegia (Table 2.5)
- Pneumonia is the most common cause of death (70%) in patients with complete or incomplete injuries
- This is followed by cardiovascular events and sepsis from decubitus ulcers, urosepsis and pneumonia

Common complications

- Pulmonary
  — aggressive pulmonary toilet
- Urinary tract infections
  — intermittent catheterization in chronic setting
- Deep vein thrombosis (DVT) and pulmonary embolism
  — immediate DVT prophylaxis and begin warfarin treatment for 2 months' duration
- Ileus is common
  — begin bowel regimes and use nasogastric tubes in acute setting
- Decubitus ulcers
  — frequent turning and reposition to relieve pressure
- Heterotopic ossification
  — begin early physical therapy and editronate
- Lack of abdominal sensation
  — evaluate for intra-abdominal injuries
- Hyperkalaemia
  — seen with administration of succinylcholine

TABLE 2.5 Life expectancy after initial hospitalization (years)				
Age at injury	Paraplegia	Low quadriplegia C5–C8	High quadriplegia C1–C4	Vent-dependent
20	45.3	40.2	35.9	16.4
40	27.7	23.5	20.0	6.9
60	12.8	10.0	7.8	1.4

TABLE 2.6 Dermatome sensory levels	
C4	Top of shoulders, sternal notch
C5	Lateral sides of upper extremities
C6	Thumb and index finger (first and second phalanges)
C–7	Middle and ring finger (third and fourth phalanges)
C8	Little finger (fifth phalange)
T1	Medial sides of upper extremities
T2,3	Anterior chest above nipples
T4	Level of nipples on chest
T5–9	Along associated intercostals space
T10	Level of umbilicus
T11,12	Lower abdomen
L1	Pubic symphysis and inguinal ligament
L2	Anterior thigh
L3	Medial knee
L4	Medial lower leg and anterior knee
L5	Lateral lower leg and great toe
S1	Fifth toe and heel
S2	Back of thigh and lateral buttocks
S3	Medial area of buttocks
S4	Perineum
S5	Perianal skin

- **Hypoxia and hypotension are the leading causes of secondary brain injury and must be avoided**
- **Do not treat hypertension in the trauma patient until traumatic brain injury is ruled out**

FURTHER READING

Bracken M B, Shepard M J, Holford T R et al 1998 Methylprednisolone or tirilazad mesylate administration after acute spinal cord injury: 1-year follow up. Results of the third National Acute Spinal Cord Injury randomized controlled trial. Journal of Neurosurgery 89(5):699–706

TABLE 2.7 Motor innervation level	
C1–4	Diaphragm, sternocleidomastoids
C5	Deltoid and biceps muscles
C6	Wrist extensors
C7	Wrist flexors
C8	Finger extensors
T1	Intrinsic hand muscles
L2	Hip flexors—psoas
L3	Knee extension—quadriceps
L4	Ankle dorsiflexion—tibialis anterior
L5	Toe dorsiflexion
S1	Ankle plantarflexion—gastrocnemius
S2	Anal sphincter tone
S3	Anal sphincter tone

Piatt J H 2005 Detected and overlooked cervical spine injury among
comatose trauma patients: from the Pennsylvania Trauma Outcomes
Study. Neurosurgical Focus 19(4):E6

Steill I G, Clement C M, McKnight R D et al 2003 The Canadian C-spine
rule versus the NEXUS low-risk criteria in patients with trauma. The New
England Journal of Medicine 349:2510–2518

Torina P J, Flanders A E, Carrino J A et al 2005 Incidence of vertebral artery
thrombosis in cervical spine trauma: correlation with severity of spinal
cord injury. AJNR American Journal of Neuroradiology 26(10):2645–2651.

Roberts I, Schierhout G, Wakai A 2005 Mannitol for acute traumatic brain
injury. Cochrane Database of Systematic Reviews 4:CD001049

NECK INJURY

PENETRATING INJURY

Background

Management of penetrating neck injury requires decisive and
accurate actions to prevent rapid deterioration. Advances in
diagnostic and interventional radiology have augmented the
sensitivity and specificity of the physical examination in detecting
injuries. As a result, an increasing number of patients are
successfully managed with selective, non-operative care.

Essentials

- 20–25% of patients with penetrating neck injury will require an
  emergency airway procedure

- Rapid assessment is essential, as expanding haematomas and soft-tissue swelling can make endotracheal intubation more difficult within minutes
- Early intubation, with the most experienced personnel available, is paramount
- Obtain a basic neurological examination (GCS, moving hands/ feet) before sedation and paralysis
  — hemiplegia may herald inadequate collateral cerebral blood flow and may greatly influence the operative decision-making process
- Hard signs (active bleeding, expanding haematomas, stridor) mandate immediate neck exploration
- Control of external bleeding is best accomplished with direct digital control by a provider wearing proper universal precautions
  — blind clamping is to be condemned
- The neck (anterior to the posterior border of the sternocleidomastoid muscle) is divided into three zones that dictate operative approach and structures at risk of injury (see Fig. 1.9)
  — zone I extends from the clavicles to the cricoid cartilage
  — zone II from the cricoid to the angle of the mandible
  — zone III extends from the angle of the mandible to the base of the skull

Resuscitation and immediate management
- Initial resuscitation follows <C>ABC principles (see Chapter 1 Resuscitation)
- Priorities include digital control of bleeding while attention is focused on establishing a secure airway
- A rapid sequence intubation technique (RSI), utilizing cricoid pressure, liberal suctioning, sedatives and paralytics, should be employed to afford the best opportunity of success on the first pass
- A trained individual should be at the head of the bed ready to perform an airway rescue technique, such as cricothyroidotomy if endotracheal intubation fails
- A surgical airway is rarely required, but when necessary should be performed without hesitation
- Fluid resuscitation should be limited to maintain a systolic blood pressure of 90 mmHg or a palpable radial pulse (see Chapter 1 Resuscitation)

Every neck wound should be thought of as a possible chest wound

Adjuncts

- Antibiotics: should cover skin flora as well as oropharyngeal organisms
- Tetanus prophylaxis

Investigation and diagnosis

Clinical evaluation

- Cervical spine immobilization in penetrating neck trauma is neither prudent nor practical
  — if in situ the collar should be removed immediately to allow complete inspection of the neck
- A full secondary examination should be performed, including inspection of the back, axilla and groin areas, to look for additional surface wounds
- Once hard signs of vascular injury have been excluded, vascular assessment proceeds with an examination for any neurological deficits
- Findings suggestive of hypopharyngeal or oesophageal penetration include
  — dysphagia
  — odynophagia
  — haemoptysis
  — haematemesis
  — subcutaneous emphysema
- Patients with laryngotracheal injury often present with obvious signs of airway injury, such as stridor, dyspnoea or subcutaneous crepitus
- Physical examination findings in the aerodigestive tract are sensitive for detecting injury but lack specificity

X-ray evaluation

- Chest radiograph (CXR) is obtained early to rule out haemopneumothoraces
  — pleural capping seen on CXR may indicate injury to the great vessels and haemorrhage into the superior mediastinum
- AP and lateral radiographs of the neck can be obtained to assist with defining trajectory of ballistic injury and to identify retained foreign bodies

Non-operative evaluation

- For haemodynamically stable patients, and those without hard signs, a diagnostic work-up should proceed to interrogate the vascular structures and aerodigestive tract (see Chapter 1 Imaging)

- For zone I injuries, angiographic evaluation of the aortic arch and its run-off vessels should be performed. If the trajectory is limited to zone II or III, angiography of the carotids and vertebrals is sufficient

- Oesophageal evaluation with oesophagoscopy and/or oesophagography should be performed in those with zone I and II involvement. Zone III evaluation of the hypopharynx is difficult at this level and injuries are frequently missed. Consider barium swallow in the awake, cooperative patient or rigid pharyngoscopy/laryngoscopy in the intubated patient

- The airway should be evaluated endoscopically (tracheobronchoscopy, diagnostic laryngoscopy, nasopharyngoscopy) in all zones

- Although formal angiography remains the gold standard, many centres are using computed tomography with angiography (CTA) or magnetic resonance angiography (MRA) for vascular evaluation

- In addition, in an effort to perform a more directed evaluation, many centres are now using CT scan to define trajectory in penetrating neck injury. This appears to be more beneficial in firearm injuries as the bullet leaves a soft-tissue path easily identified on CT scan. This often allows the elimination of some, if not all, of the standard diagnostic steps (Fig. 2.3).

> Haemodynamically abnormal patients, those with 'hard signs', and those with positive findings on aerodigestive and/or vascular evaluation should undergo surgical neck exploration

BLUNT INJURY

Background

With the exception of injuries to the cervical spine, blunt trauma results in significantly fewer injuries in the neck compared with penetrating injury. In addition to the life-threatening complications related to laryngotracheal trauma, blunt cerebrovascular injuries (BCVI) are associated with an often insidious presentation but

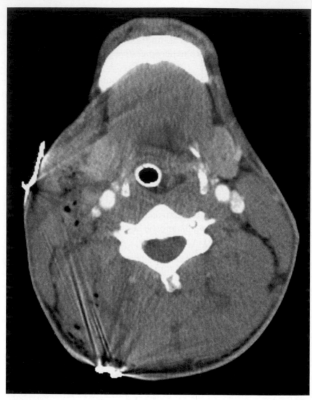

Figure 2.3 CT of the neck demonstrating gunshot wound trajectory lateral to vascular and aerodigestive structures

devastating sequelae. Although rare, blunt injuries to the cervical oesophagus are (as a result of delays in diagnosis) equally associated with significant morbidity and life-threatening complications.

Essentials
- Mechanism of injury includes direct force (seatbelt or 'clothesline' injury), hyperflexion/extension or direct compression (hanging or ligature)
- Patients sustaining blunt trauma to the neck require rapid assessment and establishment of a protected airway, as well as large-bore peripheral i.v. access

- The incidence of BCVI is less than 0.4%
  — the mortality rate of BCVI is almost 30%
  — non-lethal injuries result in significant neurological deficits in almost two-thirds of patients
  — 90% of patients with BCVI will already have neurological symptoms when the diagnosis is established
  — beware of injury patterns at high risk for BCVI
    cervical spine fractures involving C1–C3 or transverse foramen
    Le Fort II and III fractures
- Fever, tachypnoea and tachycardia may be the initial presentation of a missed aerodigestive injury

> High-risk of blunt cerebrovascular injury (>40%)
> - GCS <6
> - Petrous bone fracture
> - Diffuse axonal injury
> - LeFort II/ III fracture
> - Complex C-spine fractures with foramen transversarium involvement
> - Subluxation or injury of C1–C3

Resuscitation and immediate management
- Initial resuscitation follows <C>ABC principles (see Chapter 1 Resuscitation)
- Endotracheal intubation should be considered early *and reconsidered often*
- Personnel capable of advanced airway manoeuvres (including surgical cricothyroidotomy or tracheostomy) are required early in the resuscitation process
- A brief and focused neurological examination (including cranial nerves and extremity motor strength) should be obtained *and documented* during the initial evaluation
- Strict cervical spine immobilization (with logroll precaution and a rigid collar) should be implemented immediately and continued until definitive clearance

Investigation and diagnosis

Clinical examination
- Physical examination and secondary survey should proceed similar to that for penetrating injuries (see above)
- Careful attention should be paid to loss of the normal anatomic neck contours, the presence of subcutaneous emphysema, or

supraclavicular ecchymosis as a result of direct blunt force from the seatbelt shoulder harness
- As many patients will present with a normal initial examination, serial neurological evaluation is critical

> Patients presenting with neurological deficits and a normal CT scan of the head have a BCVI until proven otherwise

Radiographic evaluation
- CT scan of the cervical spine is more cost-effective and more reliable than plain films in the identification of cervical level fractures
- CT scan for soft tissues of the neck is helpful in identifying pretracheal oedema, subcutaneous emphysema and other signs of aerodigestive injuries
- Lateral neck films may demonstrate pretracheal soft-tissue swelling or subcutaneous emphysema
  — adds little to the evaluation of patients undergoing CT of the neck and cervical spine
- CTA can be performed simultaneously with other screening trauma CT scans.
  — experience is limited: CTA is not recommended by the centre with the largest experience in identifying BCVI, based on its insensitivity at missing minimal intimal irregularities that can lead to devastating injuries
- Duplex ultrasonography is non-invasive and reproducible, but lacks adequate sensitivity and specificity for both carotid and vertebral injuries
  — duplex is also extremely operator/technician-dependent
- MRA is a valuable screening tool in diagnosing BCVI
  — MRA produces quality images of all four vessels and is also non-invasive
- Four-vessel angiogram, although invasive and resource-consuming, *remains the gold standard* in diagnosis of BCVI
  — with appropriate screening criteria, some centres have reduced the number of unnecessary formal angiograms so that one out of three is positive for BCVI
- Evaluation of the aerodigestive tract is similar to that for penetrating injuries (see above)

Over half of patients present with initial symptoms of
BCVI 12 h or more after injury
   One-third become symptomatic 24 h or more after
sustaining trauma

Management

Operative treatment

- Surgical intervention should be reserved for those patients with
  common carotid or proximal internal carotid injuries
    — these are usually associated with significant distal dissection
      and/or pseudoaneurysm formation
- Operative approach to the vertebral artery is extremely
  limited and should be approached non-operatively or with
  interventional/endovascular assistance
- With existent neurological deficits at the time of diagnosis the
  patient should *not* undergo intervention, as the deficit is likely
  established and will only be worsened with surgery

Interventional/endovascular treatment

- Coil embolization has been used with some success in treatment
  of vertebral injuries, in light of their inability to be accessed
  surgically
- Several case reports in the literature have noted successful
  management with stent repair of carotid injuries. As with other
  endovascular applications in trauma, no large randomized studies
  have been performed and long-term follow-up is not available

Pharmacological intervention

- Patients with documented BCVI who do not receive
  anticoagulation/antiplatelet therapy have a 40–50% risk of
  developing neurological sequelae
- Early anticoagulation evaluation of patients with BCVI has been
  suggested to reduce associated neurological sequelae and should
  be the gold standard for non-operative management
- The optimal means of establishing anticoagulation remains
  controversial, as both heparinoids and antiplatelet agents have
  shown benefit

MAXILLOFACIAL INJURIES

Background

Maxillofacial injuries occur more often as a result of blunt trauma, with about 50% related to motor vehicle crashes. In car safety devices have been credited with decreasing the incidence of these injuries.

General approach to facial trauma

- The <C>ABCs take precedence over all else
- Do not be distracted by disfiguring facial injuries
  — life-threatening injuries, including an airway obscured by blood, must be treated first
- Fractured mandibles can cause obstruction of the airway
  — distract the flail segments to open the airway
- Few facial injuries are life-threatening, and delayed repair is often appropriate, but missed diagnosis can lead to poor outcomes
- Assume cervical spine injuries in patients presenting with blunt maxillofacial trauma
- All patients with open wounds require tetanus prophylaxis if not up to date

 Don't be distracted by disfiguring facial injuries!

SOFT-TISSUE FACIAL INJURIES

- Bleeding scalp lacerations can lead to exsanguination, especially in children
- Control of bleeding is part of the primary survey

 Beware the bleeding scalp laceration!

Management of face/head trauma (Table 2.8)

- Use regional anaesthesia blocks rather than local anaesthetic infiltration whenever feasible for facial wounds as there is less tissue distortion when repairing the injury
- Carefully assess areas of traumatic anaesthesia prior to administering a local or regional anaesthetic

TABLE 2.8 Sutures for the face	
Face	6/0 non-absorbable
Lip musculature	4/0 absorbable
Lip mucous membrane	4/0 or 5/0 absorbable
External lip	6/0 non-absorbable/absorbable
Buccal mucosa/nasal mucosa	4/0 absorbable
Ear	5/0 non-absorbable

- Scalp wounds can be rapidly closed with staples
- Shave the edges of scalp wounds as maximal exposure is needed
- Scalp wounds need to be closed in two layers (close the aponeurosis first)
- Perform only very limited debridement on the face
    — retain as much skin as possible
- Be aware of Langer's lines and try to repair wounds accordingly
- Facial wounds should be repaired with a 6-0 non-absorbable suture
- Lacerations across the vermilion border need special attention when being repaired
    — the human eye can perceive even the smallest error in approximation
- Be sure to examine the buccal mucosa
    — lacerations inside the mouth are often missed
- Never shave eyebrows
    — they don't always grow back!
- Know the anatomy of the facial nerve, trigeminal nerve and parotid duct
    — lacerations through each of these can lead to poor outcomes

All sutures on the face out in 5 days (10 days on the ear if cartilage involved)

Facial fractures
- Plain x-rays are adequate for many fractures, but CT imaging of the face with coronal reconstructions are becoming the standard of care
- Cerebrospinal fluid (CSF) rhinorrhoea is suggestive of a cribriform plate fracture

- CSF otorrhoea is suggestive of a temporal bone fracture
- Leakage of CSF or intracranial air on CT/x-ray indicates an open skull fracture
  — most clinicians administer prophylactic antibiotics despite the lack of prospective controlled trials
- Avoid nose blowing in facial fractures
- Patients with facial fractures should have the head of the bed elevated if feasible

Orbit fractures

- Typically fractures occur in the floor of the orbit
  — orbital roof and medial orbital wall fractures are much less common
- Mechanism is direct trauma to the eye
- Forces are transmitted to the weakest part of the orbit (the floor)
- Herniation of orbital contents (most common is inferior rectus muscle) is called a blow out fracture
- Patients present with a sunken eye with poor ocular motility
  — with or without diplopia
  — with or without infraorbital anaesthesia
- Fractures of the orbit are often associated with zygoma fractures (see below)
- Accumulation of air or blood within the bony orbit (retrobulbar haematoma) can cause stretching and hypoperfusion of the central retinal artery
  — an emergency lateral canthotomy must be performed to release this pressure

Frontal sinus

- Fractures of the anterior wall of the frontal sinus result in cosmetic deformity
- Extension into the posterior wall of the sinus indicates a dural tear
  — the patient must have the head of the bed elevated and be started on antibiotics

Maxilla

- Blood in the maxillary sinus suggests a fracture to one of the walls of the sinus
- Midface fractures are classified using the Le Fort sytem (Fig. 2.4)
- Le Fort fractures can be clinically diagnosed by examining the maxillary teeth and soft palate, as the amount of midface mobility suggests the type of fracture

— Le Fort I: motion of alveolar ridge and hard palate only
— Le Fort II: motion of the entire midface
— Le Fort III: facial structures move freely; the fracture lines essentially produce craniofacial separation

Examine all patients with nasal/midface trauma for a septal haematoma— undrained haematomas can lead to septal necrosis!

Zygoma
- Second most common facial fracture
- There are essentially two fractures of the zygoma that are seen clinically following trauma; both occur as a result of direct trauma to the region

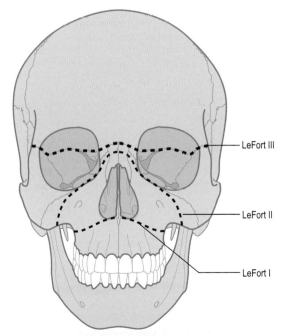

Figure 2.4 Fracture lines defining the Le Fort fractures

- Most common fracture is the tripod fracture (Fig. 2.5)
  — loss of contour of the cheek, anaesthesia of the cheek, with or without gaze abnormalities
  — zygomaticomaxillary complex is essentially separated from the remainder of the face along the fracture lines
  — tripod fractures need to be repaired urgently
- The less common zygoma fracture is a simple depression of the zygomatic arch

Nasal

- Nasal fractures are the most common facial fracture
- Rarely a problem; requires only control of bleeding and evaluation to ensure that there is no septal haematoma
- Trauma to the bridge of the nose can result in nasoethmoid fracture, with CSF rhinorrhoea suggesting dural disruption requiring further attention
- If no CSF exposure is expected, patients may undergo elective cosmetic repair

Mandible

- This is the third most common facial fracture

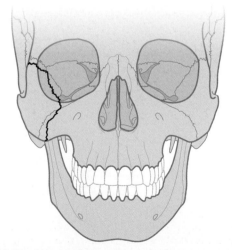

Figure 2.5 Tripod (zygomaticomaxillary complex) fractures disrupt the zygoma from the face through three fracture lines

- Fractured mandibles can cause obstruction of the airway
  — distract the flail segments to open the airway
- Patients present with pain, tenderness, malocclusion
- The mandible is essentially a circular structure
  — assume a fracture in two locations
  — fractures may be remote from the site of trauma, as forces are transmitted to the weakest part of the ring
- Most fractures occur in the angle or body of the mandible
- Assess for anaesthesia in the distribution of the inferior alveolar nerve
- Fractures involving the jaw and teeth are considered open fractures, and antibiotic prophylaxis including oral antimicrobial rinse are the standard of care

> A fractured mandible can lead to an obstructed and bloody airway—be prepared for a difficult intubation

Dental
- Adults have 32 teeth
- Paediatric patients have 20 teeth
- Subluxed teeth can be attached to adjacent teeth with arch bars, wires or bonding, and be treated conservatively with a soft diet
- Review the chest x-ray to ensure that missing teeth have not been aspirated

 Beware the missing tooth!

- Avulsed teeth should be irrigated with saline or tap water but not scrubbed
- Avulsed teeth can be replaced immediately in adults but not in children
- Teeth can be transported in commercial transport medium, milk, saline, under the tongue, or in the cheek
- Dental fractures are classified according to the Ellis classification (Fig. 2.6)
  — Ellis 1: fracture through enamel only
  — Ellis 2: fracture through enamel with exposed dentin
  — Ellis 3: fracture through enamel with exposed dentin and pulp

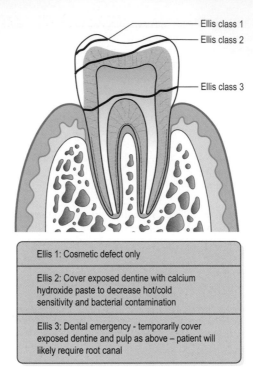

| Ellis 1: Cosmetic defect only |
| Ellis 2: Cover exposed dentine with calcium hydroxide paste to decrease hot/cold sensitivity and bacterial contamination |
| Ellis 3: Dental emergency - temporarily cover exposed dentine and pulp as above – patient will likely require root canal |

Figure 2.6 Ellis classification of dental fractures and emergency treatment

Maxillofacial trauma terms
- Battle's sign: retroauricular ecchymosis suggestive of basilar skull fracture
- Raccoon eyes: periorbital ecchymosis suggestive of basilar skull fracture
- Seidel sign: streaming of fluorescein dye with draining vitreous suggestive of a ruptured globe
- Hanging drop sign: on plain film of orbit (Water's view) evidence of extrusion of intraocular muscles (inferior rectus) through orbital floor

OPHTHALMIC INJURIES

Background

The anatomy of the orbit provides some relative protection to the eye and often allows the eye to escape injury in the severely injured patient. When injuries do occur they are frequently associated with head and facial injuries following blunt trauma. In military conflict, eye injury from fragments is fairly common because this area is relatively unprotected. Isolated eye injuries are common in industrial accidents with machine operators working with stone and metal.

> Multiply injured patients are assessed and managed in a supine position. Therefore when evaluating for ophthalmic injury the use of a slit lamp or wall-mounted Snellen chart is not possible

Essentials

- Assessment of visual function (visual acuity) should be documented in any patient with a potential eye injury
- The easiest way to perform visual acuity assessment in a supine patient is to use a visual acuity assessment tool designed for close work
- Look for significant change in visual acuity compared with normal, but remember to correct for refractive errors in those patients who normally wear visual aids
- Ophthalmic examination should proceed in a systematic fashion

OUTSIDE	→	IN
	Visual acuity	
	Pupillary responses	
	Movements	
	Lids	
	Conjunctiva/cornea	
	Anterior chamber	
	Retina	

- Do not overlook examining the eyes in a patient who is unconscious or those patients in whom the eyes are not seen due to periorbital bruising or oedema

Clinical evaluation

- Revisit the mechanism of injury, specifically thinking about blunt, penetrating, thermal or chemical injury
- Enquire about symptoms, including foreign body sensation and sudden loss of visual acuity
- Document if the patient wears glasses or contact lenses or has a significant past medical history, i.e. glaucoma
- Clinical evaluation can be performed using the following instruments
  — visual acuity assessment tool
  — bright light, blue light
  — fluorescein
  — cotton wool bud
  — blue needle

> Always remove contact lenses in unconscious patients

Goals of management for the non-specialist

- Provide analgesia—topical local anaesthesia
- Document visual function
- Remove all foreign bodies that are not embedded or penetrating
- Manage small corneal abrasions
- Manage periorbital lacerations that do not involve any significant underlying structure
- Identify associated maxillofacial fractures that may impact upon the eye, e.g. blow out fracture
- Identify patients with a significant change in visual acuity associated with sight-threatening injuries, e.g. hyphaema, vitreous haemorrhage
- Refer appropriately to ophthalmology

Common injuries and problems

Periorbital bruising/oedema

- Immediate onset of periorbital swelling/bruising usually indicates the presence of a significant facial fracture
- The eye should be gently opened and an attempt made to assess
  — visual acuity
  — pupillary responses
  — the presence of a red reflex
  — extraocular movements
- Open the eyelid with minimal pressure applied to the globe itself

- If limited initial examination reveals no obvious abnormality then re-evaluation of the eye should take place once the swelling has settled to determine whether specialist referral is required

Lacerations
- Many lacerations around the eyes can be cleaned and closed
- Horizontal superficial lacerations to the eyelid can be closed
- Specialist assessment is required for
  — deep lacerations to the eyelid that might involve the levator muscle
  — any laceration that involves or is close to the lid margin
  — injuries that could potentially involve the lacrimal ducts or the lacrimal gland itself

Foreign bodies
- Inspect the conjunctiva and cornea, and remove superficial debris and foreign bodies either by irrigation, a cotton wool bud or a hypodermic needle
- Examine for a subtarsal foreign body by everting the upper lid
- Deeply embedded or potentially penetrating foreign bodies should be removed by a specialist

Corneal abrasions
- Large corneal abrasions are usually visible when the cornea is inspected using a bright light
- Fluorescein instilled into the eye makes these abrasions more obvious when the eye is examined with a blue light
- Simple corneal abrasions can be treated with antibiotic ointment if visual acuity is not significantly impaired

Pupillary responses
- Contusion of the iris may lead to traumatic mydriasis, giving rise to a dilated unresponsive pupil
  — in the patient who has an associated head injury and altered consciousness this needs to be differentiated from a lateralizing sign
- Given the association with hyphaema, traumatic mydriasis requires specialist review

Eye movements
- Patients with double vision on examination, particularly those with obvious limitation of elevation of one eye, require CT imaging to rule out a blow out fracture
- Non-urgent referral to a specialist is required

Anterior chamber injuries

- Penetrating injuries to the anterior chamber may leave the chamber shallow and the cornea deformed
- These findings may be subtle and therefore missed by the inexperienced
- Such injuries are usually associated with a reduction in the normal visual acuity
- Specialist referral is required

Hyphaema

- Hyphaema is blood in the anterior chamber that occurs as a result of trauma to the blood vessels of the iris or ciliary body
- Presentation is typically pain and/or decreased visual acuity
- Requires urgent referral to a specialist
- Treatment may be conservative, including elevation of the head of the bed, miotics, mydriatics, cycloplegics and steroids
- Close monitoring for elevated intraocular pressure is required, as occlusion of aqueous outflow may result
- Patients are at risk for re-bleeding several days after the injury occurs when the organized clot resorbs

Globe disruption

- Disruption of the globe can occur with penetrating or blunt trauma to the eye
- Patients typically complain of eye pain and decreased vision
- Ruptures may be obvious, with a sunken eye and frank extrusion of vitreous humor, or may be occult with only subconjunctival haemorrhage apparent
- Management includes
  — avoiding further trauma (including serial examinations or tonometry)
  — emergent CT scan of the orbit
  — broad spectrum antibiotics
  — emergent ophthalmological examination with indirect ophthalmoscopy
  — urgent specialist referral

Traumatic iritis

- Typically presents with delayed aching pain several hours after traumatic injury to the eye
- Pain results from inflammation and spasm of the ciliary body
- Physical findings include ciliary flush, and '*cell and flare*' in the anterior chamber
- Patients typically improve with cycloplegic agents ± ocular steroids

Dramatic reduction in visual function
- Patients who complain of altered vision and have a reduced visual acuity need specialist assessment, particularly if the cause is not evident on external examination
- Sudden loss of vision associated with a foreign body sensation may indicate an intraocular foreign body
- Patients who have lost the red reflex may have a vitreous haemorrhage
- Patients with visual loss associated with a visual field defect need to be screened for a retinal detachment

Contact lens wearers need pseudomonal coverage

Chemical injury
- Chemical injury to the eye can be sight-threatening
- Alkalis are more dangerous than acids, though both require immediate first aid and referral
- Analgesia and prolonged irrigation to normalize the pH are the mainstays of initial management

- Always examine the eye in severely injured patients
- Although many eye injuries can be managed initially in the Emergency Department, timely specialist referral for assessment and management is important

Urgently refer:
- Traumatic mydriasis
- Hyphaema
- Extraocular muscle entrapment
- Double vision
- Decreased acuity
- Anterior chamber injuries
- Penetrating injuries

TORSO

DAMAGE CONTROL

Background

Traditionally the goal of operative intervention for injured patients was the complete identification and definitive treatment of *all* injuries in one stage. However, some severely injured patients may not tolerate a definitive procedure if performed as a single stage. The patient may have undergone a technically superb operation and yet succumb because of the duration or magnitude of the initial operation.

> Damage control is the approach of *staging* the operative care of the patient to prevent or interrupt the lethal triad of hypothermia, coagulopathy and metabolic acidosis

The stages of damage control are:

- Recognition of the need for damage control during trauma evaluation
- Control of life-threatening haemorrhage and gastrointestinal contamination
- Resuscitation in the ICU for correction of
  — acidosis
  — coagulopathy
  — hypothermia
- Return to the operating room for complete identification and definitive treatment of injuries
- Closure of wound

> The principles of damage control can be applied to injuries of the abdomen, pelvis, thorax and extremities

Stages of damage control (Fig. 2.7)

DC 0
Damage control should be a deliberate decision, based on rapid evaluation of mechanism of injury, anatomy of injury and patient physiology.

The decision to perform damage control should be made in the Trauma Resuscitation Area or *early* in the course of an operation.

Conditions for considering damage control:

- Multiple penetrating injuries to the torso
- High-energy blunt trauma to the torso
- Multisystem trauma with competing operative/interventional priorities
- Profound haemorrhagic shock at presentation

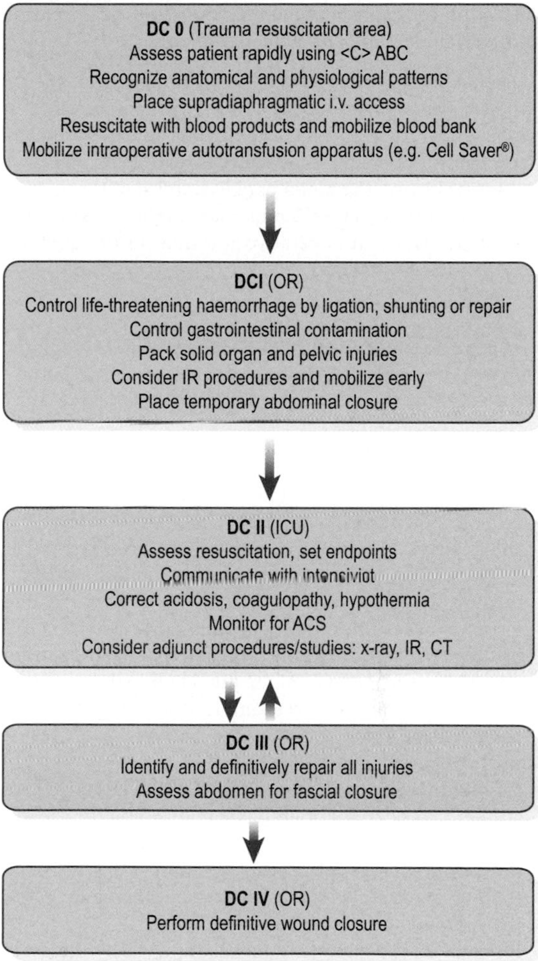

DC 0 (Trauma resuscitation area)
Assess patient rapidly using <C> ABC
Recognize anatomical and physiological patterns
Place supradiaphragmatic i.v. access
Resuscitate with blood products and mobilize blood bank
Mobilize intraoperative autotransfusion apparatus (e.g. Cell Saver®)

DCI (OR)
Control life-threatening haemorrhage by ligation, shunting or repair
Control gastrointestinal contamination
Pack solid organ and pelvic injuries
Consider IR procedures and mobilize early
Place temporary abdominal closure

DC II (ICU)
Assess resuscitation, set endpoints
Communicate with intensivist
Correct acidosis, coagulopathy, hypothermia
Monitor for ACS
Consider adjunct procedures/studies: x-ray, IR, CT

DC III (OR)
Identify and definitively repair all injuries
Assess abdomen for fascial closure

DC IV (OR)
Perform definitive wound closure

Figure 2.7 The phases of damage control. DC, damage control; OR, operating room; IR, interventional radiology; ICU, intensive care unit; ACS, abdominal compartment syndrome; CT, computed tomography

- Evidence of worsening hypothermia, coagulopathy, or metabolic acidosis on presentation or early in evaluation

The patient is rapidly evaluated by the trauma team, addressing catastrophic haemorrhage, airway control by rapid sequence intubation; intravenous access is established (preferably above the diaphragm if abdominopelvic injury is suspected); and blood is infused early. The blood bank is notified of the need for uncrossmatched blood while crossmatched blood is being prepared. If available, intraoperative autotransfusion equipment (e.g. Cell Saver®) is mobilized.

DC I

Successful implementation of damage control requires continuous coordination of care among the surgeons, anaesthetists and intensivists.

Technical considerations:

- Control exsanguinating haemorrhage quickly
  — make a generous incision and place packs into all quadrants. Explore systematically
  — shunt major arterial injuries (injuries to aorta, external iliac, and possibly superior mesenteric artery) unless primary repair is straightforward
  — ligate venous injuries (except suprarenal cava)
  — ligate smaller arteries unless primary repair is straightforward
  — strongly consider and mobilize interventional radiology for arteriography/embolization for hepatic or pelvic haemorrhage
- Control solid organ injuries
  — for liver injuries, pack, suture, ligate, coagulate
  — strongly consider arteriography/embolization for hepatic and pelvic haemorrhage
  — for splenic injuries, perform splenectomy rather than salvage
  — for high-grade renal injuries, perform nephrectomy rather than salvage
  — for high-grade pancreatic injuries, drain widely. Resect if straightforward
- Control gastrointestinal (GI) contamination
  — isolate GI contamination by rapid primary closure, umbilical tape ligation or stapling (bowel resection is optional)
  — leave the GI tract discontinuous. GI anastomoses and stomas should not be created at this time
- Terminate operation
  — leave packs in place

— leave GI tract discontinuous
— create temporary wound closure
  skin closure with suture or towel clips
  'Vac-pac' dressing: cover a theatre towel with sterile
    impervious adhesive drape (e.g. Ioban™). With smooth
    surface down, cover viscera, tucking edges under fascia
  Place two Jackson–Pratt drains along wound edges. Dry off
    surrounding skin edges and prepare with benzoin solution.
    Connect drains to high wall suction. Cover entire wound
    and surrounding skin with another Ioban™, allowing a
    vacuum to form. Do not pull Ioban™ tightly across wound.
    Maintain impervious seal
  'Bogota bag' (sterilized i.v. bag) sewn to skin
— transport to interventional radiology or surgical intensive
  care unit (SICU)

DC II

The patient undergoes resuscitation in the ICU with the goal of
rapidly assessing volume status and reversing (or preventing) the
lethal triad of hypothermia, metabolic acidosis and coagulopathy.

- Communicate with ICU team
  — define specific endpoints of resuscitation
  — measure bladder pressures (for abdominal compartment
    syndrome; ACS) and airway pressures
- Correct lethal triad
  — rewarm externally
  — infuse warmed i.v. fluids
  — ventilate with warmed gases
  — monitor intravascular volume status closely. Consider
    invasive monitoring
  — transfuse using both colloid and crystalloid, monitoring for
    signs of abdominal hypertension and ACS
  — monitor lactic acid clearance
  — perform adjunct radiographic/interventional procedures as
    indicated (x-ray, CT, interventional radiology)
- Continuously assess response to interventions

Resuscitation should be 'aggressive' in the intensity of care, which
should not be confused with overzealous fluid administration.
From a fluid balance perspective, over-resuscitation is as harmful as
under-resuscitation. Also, the presence of a temporary abdominal
closure does not rule out the possibility of ACS.

For the patient who is physiologically 'captured' (i.e. responds
appropriately to resuscitation), DC II may last between 12 and 48 h,
at which time the patient returns to the operating room for DC III.

As the patient's condition allows, adjunct studies such as x-ray, CT and interventional radiology procedures may be performed as clinically indicated.

The optimal time to return for DC III is unique to each patient.

Performing DC III prematurely may precipitate instability during the procedure and force a reversion back to DC I. Conversely, delaying DC III allows unrecognized injuries to progress, increases hollow viscera oedema and dilatation, and may increase infectious complications.

> Patients who do not respond appropriately early in the course of DC II, manifested by persistent acidosis or anaemia, should be considered to have an uncontrolled source of haemorrhage and return to the operating room or the interventional radiology suite to exclude surgical bleeding

DC III

The patient returns to the operating room for a thorough evaluation, identification and definitive treatment of injuries.

- Assess injuries carefully and thoroughly
  — resect necrotic tissue, remove clots
  — perform GI anastomoses and stomas
  — perform autologous vein or prosthetic bypass grafts
  — assess wound for definitive closure

If definitive wound closure is not possible, another temporary wound closure is placed, and the patient returns to the ICU for ongoing care. The wound is frequently re-evaluated for closure.

GI anastomoses are at an increased risk of leak, and it is probably helpful to 'bury' these deeper within the abdominal cavity so that they are not exposed in a wound which will require repeated inspections. Similarly, although long-term enteral access (gastrostomy and jejunostomy tubes) is sometimes desirable, the complication rate is probably higher, and these should be performed with caution in patients who require repeated inspections of the abdomen.

Tubes, drains and stomas should be brought out lateral to the rectus sheath, preserving it for possible future use in abdominal wall reconstruction.

DC IV

Many options exist for definitive wound closure:

- Primary fascial closure with or without skin closure
- Fascial closure with mesh
- Skin closure only, with fascial defect
- Split thickness skin graft
- Serial fascial approximation aided by prosthetic sheets (e.g. Wittmann Patch™) or negative pressure therapy (e.g. VAC®)
- Reconstruction by component separation

Patients who undergo skin grafting of the open abdomen may return after several months for complex abdominal wall reconstruction.

Perils and pitfalls of damage control

Damage control is a deliberate strategy, not a 'bail-out'. Think about damage control early, before onset of the lethal triad.

Some sources of haemorrhage are more amenable to angioembolization than surgical ligation. Strongly consider immediate postoperative arteriography and embolization for hepatic and pelvic/retroperitoneal haemorrhage.

After multiple trips to the operating room, pack counts may be incorrect. Prior to definitive closure of the abdomen, consider intraoperative abdominal x-ray to confirm absence of laparotomy packs.

Temporary abdominal closure does not rule out ACS. Maintain awareness of recurrent ACS and check bladder pressures during resuscitation.

Control of surgical bleeding in DC I is sometimes incomplete. Suspect surgical bleeding in patients who do not respond appropriately to resuscitation.

The time required for physiological 'capture' varies from patient to patient. Do not perform DC III prematurely.

BLUNT THORACIC TRAUMA

Background

- Blunt thoracic injury accounts for about 8% of all trauma admissions in North America, and chest trauma (blunt and penetrating) accounts for one of every four trauma deaths
- Many of these patients die after reaching the hospital, and many of these deaths could be prevented with prompt diagnosis and treatment

- Given the much lower frequency of penetrating trauma in the UK, the percentage of blunt injury is significantly higher
- Motor vehicle collisions are the most common aetiology
- In children under the age of three years, child abuse is the most common cause of thoracic trauma, representing up to 66% of cases
- Given the high density of vital structures in the chest, blunt thoracic trauma has a high likelihood of causing life-threatening injury
- The trauma practitioner must be alert to the myriad of possible injuries that can occur, and competent in their treatment as recognition and treatment can be life-saving (Table 2.9)

> The chest is a target-rich environment and there are a lot of potential ways to die from chest injuries

Diagnostic techniques
- Must *complement* and *not interfere* with resuscitation
- A portable supine chest x-ray (CXR) is the standard of care for all blunt trauma patients
- Constant re-evaluation is required
- Ultrasound: excellent for pericardial effusion, and of questionable efficacy for diagnosing haemothorax or pneumothorax
- CTA is the current screening procedure of choice for aortic injury and has all but replaced angiography in most centres

TABLE 2.9 The deadly dozen blunt injuries of the chest	
The fearsome five*	*The serious seven†*
1. Airway obstruction	1. Simple pneumothorax
2. Tension pneumothorax	2. Haemothorax
3. Flail chest	3. Pulmonary contusion
4. Massive haemothorax	4. Tracheobronchial disruption
5. Cardiac tamponade	5. Blunt cardiac injury
	6. Traumatic aortic disruption
	7. Traumatic diaphragmatic injury

*Emergent, immediately life-threatening injuries that must be identified as part of the primary survey. Open pneumothorax was excluded from this list as it is uncommon in blunt thoracic trauma. †Injuries that have a high potential to be life-threatening in a delayed fashion and should be found on secondary survey

- Angiography is indicated to evaluate presumed injury to other vessels in the chest, to plan for repair of aortic injuries and may also be used in a therapeutic fashion (intravascular stents)
- Endoscopy and/or bronchoscopy are indicated for suspected injuries to airway and oesophagus

Airway injuries/airway obstruction
- A priority in all trauma patients is to ensure an adequate airway
- Blunt injury to the cervical trachea occurs in less than 1% of all patients with trauma to the trunk
- Many airway injuries can be treated non-operatively, but this can result in airway obstruction, requiring a surgical airway

CHEST WALL INJURIES
Rib fractures
- Rib fractures are the most common chest wall injury resulting from blunt trauma
- They are a marker of significant associated injuries
- Associated with morbidity secondary to pain, atelectasis and underlying pulmonary contusion
  — risk of splenic injury increased 1.7 fold with rib fracture
  — risk of hepatic injury increased 1.4 fold with rib fracture
  — first rib fractures are associated with heart and great vessel injuries in up to 15%, and head and neck injuries in up to 50% of cases
- More than three rib fractures are associated with increase in abdominal injury and mortality
- Rib fractures are less common in children, but pulmonary contusion is more common
- Mortality is higher in the elderly (five times the rate of younger patients)
- Treatment is analgesia and adequate pulmonary toilet

Flail chest
- A flail chest is the fracture of three or more consecutive ribs in two or more places, and is the most serious of the common blunt chest wall injuries (Fig. 2.8).
- This results in an incomplete segment of chest wall that is large enough to impair the patient's respiration
- The chest wall will move paradoxically on respiration with a flail chest
- High association of underlying pulmonary contusion

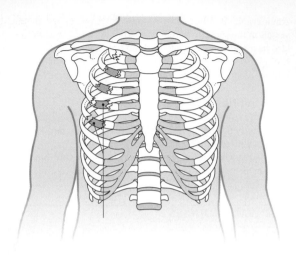

Figure 2.8 A flail chest is characterized by three or more consecutive ribs fractured in two or more places. This results in paradoxical motion

- In patients with flail chest and pulmonary contusion, 75% require ventilation and mortality rates are as high as 40%
- Treatment hinges on adequate pain control (nerve blocks, epidural analgesia and intravenous narcotics) and aggressive respiratory care
- Operative repair does *not* have wide support

Scapular fractures
- These are uncommon injuries as great force is required
- Associated injuries to lung, great vessels, brachial plexus and central nervous system are common and must be considered
- Treatment is generally non-operative and consists of immobilization

Sternal fractures
- Associated injuries are common and a high index of suspicion should be maintained for underlying visceral injuries (cardiac injury in 18–62%)
- If unstable or displaced by more than 1 cm, they should be treated with open reduction and internal fixation

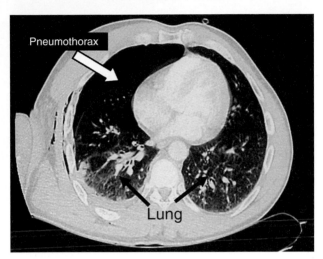

Figure 2.9 A CT scan showing partial collapse of the right lung with a simple pneumothorax

Pneumothorax

Simple pneumothorax

- A simple pneumothorax is a non-expanding collection of air between the outside surface of the lung and the inside surface of the chest wall
- Occurs in up to 24% of patients with blunt trauma
- A CXR is usually diagnostic but may miss small pneumothoraces
- The presence of rib fractures should prompt a careful search for pneumothorax
- CT is much more sensitive, but the significance of small 'occult' pneumothoraces is unknown (Fig. 2.9)
- Most simple pneumothoraces will require placement of a chest tube as definitive treatment
- Small pneumothoraces (those <20%) may be watched expectantly, unless the patient is to undergo positive pressure ventilation or will be placed in a situation where close monitoring is not possible

Tension pneumothorax

- Progressive build-up of air within the pleural space where air escapes but does not return (one-way valve effect)

- The mediastinum becomes pushed to the opposite hemithorax, with circulatory instability and eventual arrest (Fig. 2.10)
- The cause of preventable death in up to 16% of cases in the field
- *This is not an x-ray diagnosis*—if you wait for an x-ray your patient may die!
- Classic signs are deviation of the trachea, distended neck veins and hyperexpanded chest with increased percussion
- *Distended neck veins may be absent if the patient is in haemorrhagic shock*
- Immediate management is needle decompression, with a large-bore intravenous cannula placed into the second rib space at the midclavicular line above the rib
- Chest tube placement is the definitive treatment

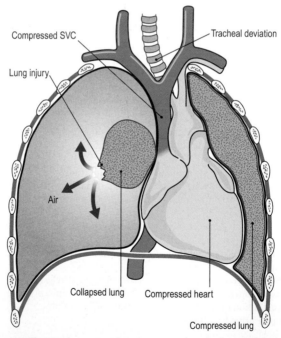

Figure 2.10 A tension pneumothorax occurs as a result of accumulation of air that can not escape in the pleural space. This causes collapse of the lung, and shifting and compression of the mediastinal structures with resultant cardiac collapse. SVC, superior vena cava

- *Tension pneumothorax can develop with a chest tube in place*
- Large persistent air leaks may require additional tubes, and usually represent injury to a major airway and a need for surgical repair

Haemothorax (one of the serious seven)

- Haemothorax is a collection of blood in the pleural space (Fig. 2.11)
- Most haemothoraces are a result of rib fractures, lung parenchyma, and minor venous injuries, and are therefore usually self-limiting
- Small haemothoraces are not detected by physical examination or CXR as it takes approximately 300 cm^3 of blood to show up on an x-ray
- Focused assessment with sonography for trauma (FAST) has success in identifying smaller haemothoraces but is very user-dependent
- CT is very sensitive for finding small amounts of blood but this may not be clinically significant
- Chest tube placement (at least 36-French) is the first step in management and is definitive in up to 90% of cases

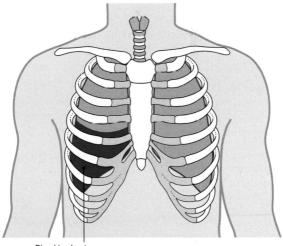

Blood in chest

Figure 2.11 Haemothorax occurs from bleeding within the thoracic cavity with layering of the blood in the chest

Massive haemothorax
- Massive haemothorax has been variably defined as more than 1000–1500 cm^3
- Clinically it is enough blood loss that the patient becomes haemodynamically unstable
- Massive haemothorax is usually a result of injury to large intrathoracic vessels or, on occasion, the heart. It can also occur from intra-abdominal bleeding in the presence of a diaphragmatic injury
- Tension haemothorax can occur with large amounts of blood present
- Classic clinical signs include shock, unilateral absence of breath sounds, dullness to percussion and flat neck veins
- Initial management is chest tube with operative exploration if indicated (see below)
- *Blood from chest tubes can be autotransfused*

Indications for urgent thoracotomy for haemorrhage
- The key here is not to wait too long in someone who really needs operative control
- If 1500 cm^3 of blood drain initially or more than 200 cm^3 per hour in the next 4 h, operative intervention is warranted
- The focus of thoracotomy for haemorrhage is
  — stop bleeding at the source
  — allow the lung to fully expand and provide tamponade
- Operative intervention may range from simple suture repair to wedge resection, staple tractotomy, lobectomy and ultimately pneumonectomy

Pericardial tamponade
- Pericardial tamponade results from accumulation of blood around the heart; this interferes with cardiac filling and restricts cardiac activity
- Relatively small amounts of blood (100 cm^3) will cause tamponade, and removal of small amounts (15–20 cm^3) may be enormously beneficial
- Diagnosis is best made by FAST, which is very sensitive for fluid in the pericardial sac (Fig. 2.12)
- Clinical diagnosis is difficult but classically includes muffled heart sounds, distended neck veins and pulsus paradoxus
- Aetiology in trauma patients is usually from a penetrating wound but can also occur in blunt trauma from cardiac rupture
- Blunt cardiac rupture is immediately fatal in >90%, and survivors usually have atrial injuries

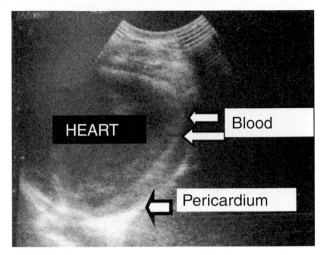

Figure 2.12 A FAST ultrasound from the pericardial position depicting fluid (blood) between the pericardium and the heart

- Definitive therapy is surgery with haemorrhage control, but pericardiocentesis and pericardial window can be diagnostic and temporizing

Pulmonary contusion
- Pulmonary contusion results from blunt injury to the lung, with bleeding into the parenchyma that can interfere with oxygenation (Fig. 2.13)
- Arguably the most common life-threatening blunt chest injury with a reported mortality rate of 5–30%
- Treatment is largely supportive, and includes oxygen, restrictive fluid resuscitation and intubation with lung protective strategies
- Unilateral contusion may benefit from split (or independent) lung ventilation

Tracheobronchial disruption
- 1–3% of motor vehicle collision victims sustain this injury
- 80% die before reaching hospital
- May result in tension pneumothorax
- Typically present with mediastinal and deep cervical emphysema, persistent air leak and pneumothorax in spite of chest tube

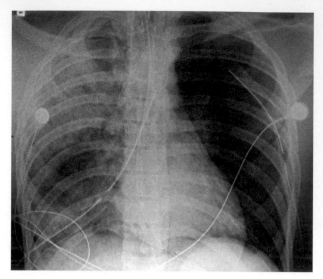

Figure 2.13 Pulmonary contusion is seen on this CXR as haziness in the right lung fields

- Most common location is within 2.5 cm of the carina, right more frequently than left
- Initial management is placement of an endotracheal tube beyond the injury, with CT scan and bronchoscopy to delineate location
- Operative repair by thoracic surgeon using incision dictated by the location of injury

Blunt cardiac injury

- The incidence of blunt cardiac injury (contusion) is 10–20%, and most cases are asymptomatic
- A small percentage (1–2%) will develop symptoms (arrhythmias or pump failure) requiring treatment
- If the ECG is normal on admission and 4 h later, the risk of life-threatening arrhythmias is nil
- *Enzymes are not indicated.* They do not predict risk of complications
- If ECG is positive, obtain a formal echocardiogram
- Bundle branch blocks may require temporary pacer
- Intra-aortic balloon pump may be required for low cardiac output
- Serious damage to virtually every cardiac structure has been reported

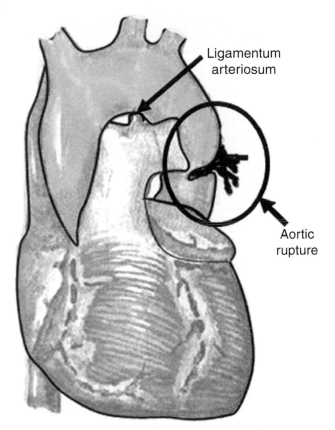

Figure 2.14 Aortic rupture classically occurs just beyond the ligamentum arteriosum. The angiogram over shows the classic picture of a contained rupture

Traumatic aortic disruption
- Deceleration and traction are the classic mechanisms; the point of fixation being the ligamentum arteriosum (Fig. 2.14)
- 70–80% of patients die at the scene
- 2–5% are unstable on presentation or rapidly become unstable; these patients have a mortality rate of 90–98%
- 25% will be stable with the diagnosis made 4–18 h after injury, with a mortality rate of around 25%, which is largely due to associated injuries

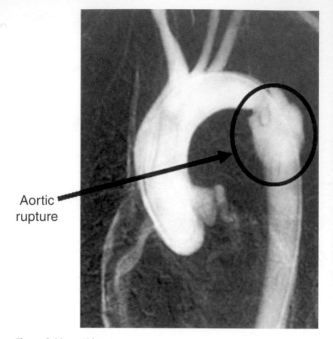

Aortic rupture

Figure 2.14 *cont'd*

- Diagnosis is suggested by following findings on CXR
  — widened mediastinum (>0.4 of the thoracic diameter)
    (Fig. 2.15)
  — loss of aortic knob
  — apical cap (blood on top of the lung)
  — loss of paraspinous stripe
  — obscured aortopulmonary window
  — nasogastric tube shifted to the right
  — left mainstem bronchus is depressed
- *A negative x-ray does not exclude aortic injury.* If clinical
  suspicion is high proceed with further studies
- Helical CTA has become the diagnostic procedure of choice,
  with 100% sensitivity, 99.7% specificity and 100% negative
  predictive value (Fig. 2.16)
- Angiography (the historic gold standard) has 100% sensitivity
  and 98% specificity. This may be useful in planning surgical
  approach, ruling out other vascular injury; it may also be
  potentially therapeutic (endovascular stent placement)

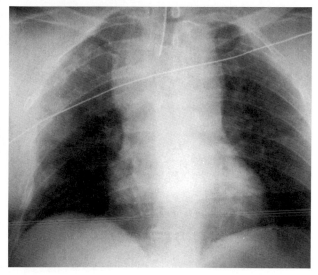

Figure 2.15 This chest x-ray depicts a widened mediastinum which should prompt helical CT

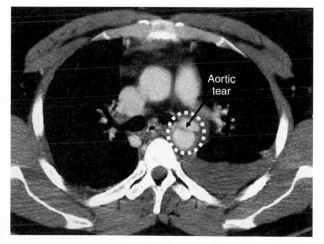

Figure 2.16 This helical CT shows a tear in the thoracic aorta just after the ligamentum arteriosum

- Initial management includes blood pressure control (<120 mmHg systolic) with beta blockers if needed, and operative repair (in 30–50%) of other life-threatening injuries
- Operative repair is best accomplished via a fourth interspace posterolateral approach with aortic control proximal to the subclavian
- Several different techniques of operative repair have been reported to include both direct suture repair and placement of a prosthetic graft
- Most feared complications of repair are paraplegia and renal failure from ischaemia
- Various methods of bypass have been shown to decrease but not to eliminate ischaemic injury

Traumatic diaphragmatic disruption
- Relatively rare (~3% of total injuries)
- 80–90% are a result of motor vehicle crashes
- 80–100% of patients with this injury will have other associated severe injuries
- Diagnosis may not be obvious and in 10–50% of cases the diagnosis is not made in the first 24 h
- CXR is helpful to determine the most common findings of elevated hemidiaphragm, bowel pattern in the chest, or a nasogastric tube passing into the abdomen and then curling up in the chest. However, CXR can be normal in up to 50% of cases
- Surgical repair is indicated even for small tears
- Early deaths are usually a result of the associated injuries, with mortality rates ranging from 5 to 30%

Complications of chest trauma
- Pneumonia is the most common complication
- Retained haemothorax leads to increased risk of empyema
- Persistent air leak with the development of a bronchopleural fistula
- Empyema usually requires operative drainage
- Lung abscess
- Pneumatocoele
- Chylothorax is uncommon

FURTHER READING

www.trauma.org/thoracic January 2007
www.aic.cuhk.edu.hk/web8/chest_injuries.htm January 2007

Karmy-Jones R, Jurkovich G J 2004 Blunt chest trauma. Current Problems in
    Surgery 41(3):211–380

PENETRATING CHEST INJURY

Background

Chest trauma contributes significantly to mortality and morbidity
rates of the injured patient (25% deaths). Immediate causes of
death include injuries to the great vessels and heart, while early
causes are attributable to airway injury, tension pneumothorax
or tamponade. Late causes of death include respiratory failure
from pulmonary contusion and sepsis. Prompt identification of
trajectory and recognition of anatomic injury, combined with
appropriate resuscitation and urgent surgical intervention (when
indicated), are the cornerstones of management. However, almost
90% of these injuries can be managed simply with appropriate chest
drain placement, aggressive pain control, and serial investigations
and monitoring.

Essentials

- Identify the patient's physiology (stable, unstable, extremis) early
  on to expedite their triage and potential intervention
- In firearm injuries, promptly obtain a chest radiograph (with
  wounds marked) to allow early estimation of trajectory
- Penetrating cardiac injuries are associated with a mortality rate
  in excess of 75%
- Stab wound depth is difficult to determine, with variable blade
  depths and unknown amount of penetration (beware the 'hilt
  sign')
- Impalement injuries are often related to falls and industrial
  mishaps, often presenting with difficulties in transport and
  evaluation (often impaled on fixed object)
- Diaphragm injuries are easily missed by CT, as well as by
  diagnostic peritoneal lavage (DPL) and FAST

 Do not probe wounds!!!

Resuscitation and immediate management

- Initial resuscitation follows <C>ABC principles (see Chapter 1
  Resuscitation)

- Tension pneumothorax is a clinical diagnosis and requires immediate decompression with a large bore cannula inserted into the second intercostal space in the midclavicular line. This should be followed by formal chest drainage with tube thoracostomy
- Haemopneumothorax may cause severe physiological disturbance and, once identified, should be drained immediately
- Cautious resuscitation and volume replacement should be undertaken to restore the patient's systolic pressure to approximately 80 mmHg
- Resuscitation should occur simultaneously with a rapid search for the source of haemorrhage

 Do not get distracted by an impaling object, no matter how impressive. The <C>ABCs remain the priority

Investigation and diagnosis

Clinical evaluation

- Quickly determine if the wound involves the pericardial 'box of death'" as these wounds will frequently require exploration (pericardial window, etc.)
- Knives and other impaling objects should be left in situ during the initial evaluation and management
- Chest tube placement can be both diagnostic and therapeutic
- Many signs of chest trauma can be detected clinically and these must be acted upon immediately
- The patient in extremis needs appropriate intervention, not a radiograph
- Beck's triad (raised CVP, hypotension, muffled heart tones) is present in less than one-third of patients
- Massive surgical emphysema of the chest and neck/face and continued massive air leak should raise suspicion of a perforation of the airway or oesophagus

Removal of retained weapons should take place under controlled conditions in the operating theatre, where vascular control can be obtained and associated damage can be dealt with appropriately

Laboratory evaluation
- The majority of laboratory values obtained in the acute setting will provide little, if any, guidance to the work-up and management of patients with penetrating chest injuries
- The only value likely to be of any benefit is a type and screen (type and cross)

Radiographic evaluation
- The trauma CXR (upright if possible) is the mainstay of diagnosis in resuscitation, and serves as a good initial screening investigation for identifying life-threatening injuries and estimating trajectory
- Additional radiographs should be obtained (or a CT scout film) to identify any and all ballistic fragments (foreign body + wounds = even number)
- Owing to the curvature of the diaphragm, there usually need to be at least 300 ml of blood present in the pleural space before it is visible on the chest radiograph, and it takes at least 500 ml to flatten the costophrenic angle on one side
- In those patients who are haemodynamically stable, CT remains the test of choice
- The strength of CT lies in defining trajectory, its weaknesses in identifying injury to the diaphragm

Number of ballistic fragments plus number of wounds (marked by paper clips) should be an *even* number. If the number is *odd*:
1. A wound is being missed
2. A ballistic fragment has not been found
3. The patient has been shot by firearm previously

FAST evaluation
- Valuable for triage of the pleural cavities for the detection of blood in unstable patients, as well as for rapid identification of free fluid in the abdomen and pericardial fluid
- Blood above and below the diaphragm indicates a diaphragm injury
- Accurate for the detection of cardiac tamponade and, with a normal CXR, can rule out cardiac injury
- This modality is less accurate than CT and is, more than other interventions, extremely operator-dependent. In addition, its accuracy and sensitivity are lower in the obese and in patients with significant amounts of subcutaneous emphysema

> Pericardiocentesis is unreliable as both a diagnostic and
> therapeutic modality and should not delay definitive
> treatment

Management

General
- Penetrating injuries to the lung parenchyma will usually cause self-limiting bleeding unless a major intrapulmonary vessel has been injured
- Haemopneumothoraces vary in size; the majority can be treated with simple chest drainage and conservative measures
- Injury to the internal mammary or intercostal vessels may result in a significant haemothorax or ongoing bleed from the chest drain; this may require definitive surgery
- Massive haemothorax is usually defined as more than 1500 ml blood out of the chest tube; the decision to perform definitive or surgical intervention depends on the rate of drainage

Thoracotomy
- Trauma thoracotomies should not be performed outside the operating theatre unless absolutely necessary
- Although there is no absolute guide to intervention for haemothorax, and clinical condition must be weighed up against the rate of drainage (i.e. whether it is increasing or decreasing), the following is a guide to indication for thoracotomy:
  — initial chest tube output greater than 1500 ml
  — >200 ml/h for 5 consecutive hours
  — >300 ml/h for 4 consecutive hours
  — >400 ml/h for 3 consecutive hours
  — >500 ml/h for 2 consecutive hours
- Other indications for thoracotomy after penetrating chest trauma include: cardiac tamponade, acute physiological deterioration, great vessel injury noted on angiogram or massive air leak
- Bronchial injuries presenting with massive air leak can often be managed with careful placement of additional chest drains to allow lung expansion. Bronchoscopy can be used to define the injury
- If the patient has arrested or is peri-arrest, an emergency thoracotomy must be performed to relieve the tamponade (see below)

- In all other patients with suspected tamponade, every effort should be made to get to the operating theatre for an urgent thoracotomy; this includes patients who are clearly in tamponade but are only slowly deteriorating
- Control of rapid haemorrhage is the first priority and the approach/positioning is of the utmost importance (to minimize any compromise to optimal exposure)

Thoracoscopy/laparoscopy

- Although of proven *diagnostic* benefit in thoracoabdominal stab wounds, therapeutic use of thoracoscopy in the acute setting is minimal
- However, as retained blood in the chest is at high risk of becoming infected and creating an empyema, many authors advocate thoracoscopic evacuation in the first several days following injury

Adjuncts

- Following an adequate primary survey and prior to departure from the emergency/trauma area, large bore peripheral access should be established and blood should be sent for a type and cross
- Rapid transport to an immediately available, pre-evaluated, properly equipped operating room is paramount
- The patient should be sterilely prepped and draped from the neck to the knees, and down to the table on both flanks
- Adequate analgesia will prevent the shallow breathing caused by pain and facilitate better tissue oxygenation
- Early antibiotics may reduce the incidence of pneumonia and empyema following penetrating chest injury
- Echocardiography can be used *postoperatively* to detect intracardiac injuries such as atrial or ventricular septal defects, chordae tendinae rupture or valvular injuries
- Bronchoscopy may be indicated if there is suspicion of major airway damage (trachea or main bronchi)
- Significant tissue loss of the chest wall may result from high energy transfer wounds. These may require soft tissue/myocutaneous coverage techniques and combined approaches with plastic surgeons

FURTHER READING

Mahoney P F, Ryan J, Brooks A J, Schwab C W (eds) 2005 Ballistic trauma. A practical guide. Springer-Verlag, Frankfurt.

EMERGENCY DEPARTMENT THORACOTOMY (EDT)

Definition
Left anterolateral thoracotomy rapidly converted to a 'clam shell' performed in the emergency department shortly after patient's arrival in an attempt to salvage a life in extremis or with recent loss of vital signs.

Background
Which patients should be subjected to this procedure has been the subject of much debate. The risk-to-benefit ratio and ethics of this procedure given the high mortality rates are often the subject of analysis. There is a cost to the institution and a resultant cost to the patient/their family, a cost to the healthcare team with use of time and resources as well as the everpresent threat of bloodborne pathogen transmission. There is also a cost to society when neurological sequelae occur in the surviving population. This procedure tends to be performed in haste and, as such, carries a higher than usual rate of viral transmission.

Survival rates and outcome
The overall survival rate for patients undergoing EDT is 7.8%. However, of those who survive, an estimated 15% will have neurological impairment. In penetrating injury, the survival rate is 11%, in blunt injury 1.6% (Table 2.10). The highest survival rates are in those patients undergoing EDT for penetrating cardiac injury, yielding a survival rate of approximately 30%. Overall survival rates are slightly higher in the paediatric population.

Recommendations for patient selection
- Blunt trauma
  EDT should be performed in patients only if the patient arrives with vital signs and then experiences a witnessed cardiopulmonary arrest

Signs of life
1. Spontaneous movements
2. Pupillary response, eye movement
3. Spontaneous respirations
4. Electrical complexes on ECG>40 beats/min

- Penetrating trauma
- EDT should be performed if

TABLE 2.10 Survival following emergency department thoracotomy	
Mechanism	*Survival*
Blunt	1.6%
Penetrating	11%

— patient arrives with vital signs and then experiences a cardiopulmonary arrest
— patient has vital signs in the field but loses them en route ±5 min
— patient has signs of life in the field or in the trauma centre but loses them

Procedure

Equipment

- Universal precautions should be used at all times
- A prepared sterilized instrument tray should be on standby at all times as long as a competent surgeon is able to perform EDT

Instruments
Scalpel with No. 22 blade
Rib spreader (large)
Large chest wall retractor ×2
Mayo scissors ×2 (short and long)
Metzenbaum scissors (long)
Aortic crossclamp
Satinski vena cava clamp
DeBakey forceps ×2
Toothed forceps ×2
Curved clamps ×4
Gigli saw with blade
Fine needle holder ×2
Internal defibrillation paddles
Sutures: 2.0 Prolene and 2.0 Vicryl
Ties: 2.0 Vicryl
Laparotomy packs
Pledgets (if available)

- This procedure should never be performed by an untrained team of healthcare providers
- The emergency department staff should be on standby to obtain extra needed equipment as well as preparing the defibrillator for use

Technique
1. The patient's entire anterior and lateral thoracic area is splash-prepped, from clavicles to the subcostal margin
2. A left anterolateral thoracotomy is performed just below the level of the left nipple (male) or inframammary fold (female) from the edge of the sternum to the latissimus dorsi at the level of the trolley. The incision is carried through the intercostal muscles, ignoring the internal mammary artery at first. A large rib spreader is inserted
3. The pericardium is opened anterior to the phrenic nerve and any haemopericardium is evacuated. The myocardium is examined for repairable injury
4. The incision is continued into a right thoracotomy —clam shell
5. If myocardial injury is found, a finger is placed over it for tamponade and it is repaired with 2/0 polypropylene suture; pledgets are preferred
6. If the heart is fibrillating, defibrillation is attempted with internal paddles ($20\rightarrow30$ J); the advanced cardiac life support (ACLS) protocol is initiated
7. If the heart is not beating, internal cardiac massage is performed; ACLS protocol is initiated
8. If the thoracic aorta is bleeding, it is compressed and clamped with a side-biting vascular clamp
9. If the pulmonary parenchyma is bleeding massively or a pulmonary hilar injury is suspected, the hilum is clamped or the inferior pulmonary ligament released and a 180° rotation of the lung is performed to tamponade the vessels around the bronchus
10. If no repairable thoracic injury is found and a palpable carotid pulse is obtained in a short time with thoracic aortic crossclamping, the patient is moved to the operating theatre for repair of infradiaphragmatic injuries

Operating room
A dedicated operating room with staff must be on standby in the event that circulation is restored. Staff must be prepared to place the patient on cardiopulmonary bypass (if available) and must also have equipment available for extended thoracic/abdominal and neck incision.

The anaesthesia staff must be prepared to assist with one-lung ventilation if necessary, and have resources for ongoing massive resuscitation available.

FURTHER READING

Practice management guidelines for emergency department thoracotomy, working group, ad hoc subcommittee on outcomes, American College of Surgeons—Committee on Trauma 2001 Journal of the American College of Surgeons 193(3):303–309

Pryor J P, Schwab C W, Peitzman A B 2001 Thoracic vascular injury. In: Peitzman A B, Rhodes M, Schwab C W et al (eds) The trauma manual 2nd edn. Lippincott Williams and Wilkins, Philadelphia, p 224–236

BLUNT ABDOMINAL TRAUMA

Background

The vast majority of blunt abdominal injuries are the result of motor vehicle crashes. Intra-abdominal injuries (IAI) are the result of compression or crush, abrupt shearing forces as a result of rapid deceleration, and acute and sudden rises in intra-abdominal pressure. More than any other region of the body, advances in diagnostic imaging and careful observation have allowed non-operative management of a significant proportion of solid organ injuries.

Essentials

- As many injuries are often predictable, accurate information regarding the mechanism of injury is important
- 50% of patients with IAI have no external signs of trauma
- *Serial* abdominal examinations are invaluable
- The true utility of FAST examination is in triaging body cavities (chest vs. abdominal vs. pericardial) as a source of hypotension
- In those patients who are haemodynamically stable, CT is the test of choice
- Diaphragm injuries are easily missed by CT, as well as by DPL and FAST

Resuscitation and immediate management

- Initial resuscitation follows <C>ABC principles (see Chapter 1 Resuscitation)
- In the patient who presents with haemodynamic instability, or those requiring ongoing fluid resuscitation, a rapid assessment of the abdomen is mandatory
- Evaluation and exposure of the patient may identify evidence of potential injury (peritoneal signs, abdominal distension) and ongoing blood loss (delayed capillary refill, decreased level of consciousness, pale and cool extremities)

- Both FAST and DPL are useful in establishing, or ruling out, the abdominal cavity as a potential source for *haemodynamic abnormalities*

> Patients who remain hypotensive or labile in the presence of positive FAST or DPL findings should undergo immediate laparotomy

Investigation and diagnosis

Clinical evaluation
- Concomitant head or spinal cord trauma, distracting extremity injuries and clinical intoxication often make the abdominal examination unreliable
- However, in the alert, awake patient, focused serial abdominal examinations (preferably performed by the same individual) are invaluable for the detection of abdominal injury

Laboratory evaluation
- The majority of laboratory values obtained in the acute setting will provide little, if any, guidance to the work-up and management of the patient with blunt abdominal trauma
- In patients who are to undergo CT scan (regardless of the laboratory results) the only values likely to be of any benefit are a type and screen (or type and crossmatch)
- The use of laboratory values, such as haemoglobin–haematocrit and amylase–lipase, are in following those patients (serially) with established intra-abdominal injuries (i.e. hepatic, splenic, pancreatic)

Radiographic evaluation
- CXR is likely to be the only plain film of any value in the evaluation of blunt abdominal trauma. A CXR, especially with a nasogastric tube in place, may help to identify an elevated or disrupted hemidiaphragm
- Abdominal plain films in *blunt* trauma are of little, if any, value
- Pelvic plain films are of benefit as a triage tool in those patients who arrive haemodynamically abnormal
  — they may help in identifying, or ruling out, a fracture pattern with potential for haemodynamically significant blood loss
- In the haemodynamically stable patient, CT of the abdomen/ pelvis remains the preferred method of evaluation for patients sustaining blunt abdominal trauma

- Weaknesses of CT in identifying IAI include hollow viscus injury and injury to the diaphragm and pancreas

FAST
- Ultrasound is non-invasive, inexpensive and easily repeated
- FAST has quickly replaced DPL as the tool of choice in the triage of hypotensive patients
- The utility of FAST in the acutely injured patient is the rapid identification of free fluid in the abdomen and pericardial fluid
- This modality is less accurate than CT and can be operator-dependent
- Accuracy and sensitivity are lower in the obese and in patients with significant amounts of subcutaneous emphysema

DPL
- DPL is an established method of identifying intra-abdominal injury following blunt abdominal trauma
- A catheter is initially passed into the peritoneal cavity and aspiration of blood or bowel contents is attempted. If this is negative for 10 ml or greater of blood or any succus, a litre of warmed normal saline is infused and the bag is then placed to gravity
- Traditional criteria for a positive lavage include: >100 000 red blood cells/mm^3, >500 white blood cells/mm^3, the presence of bacteria, succus or food particles
- DPL value is in identifying haemodynamically significant blood loss in the hypotensive trauma patient
- Many centres now simply use the initial aspirate (gross blood or succus) to determine whether or not the patient warrants laparotomy or should undergo further diagnostic work-up

> As mortality rates increase with operative delays, laboratory and other diagnostic testing should not delay operative intervention in the patient who is hypotensive or demonstrating evidence of haemodynamic deterioration

Management

Laparotomy
- Exploratory laparotomy is indicated in those hypotensive patients presenting following blunt trauma with high probability of IAI based on physical examination, FAST or DPL

- Patients with high grade splenic injury, complex hepatic injuries and suspicion of hollow viscus injury should be considered for laparotomy

Laparoscopy
- Although of proven *diagnostic* benefit in anterior abdominal stab wounds and in haemodynamically stable patients with tangential gunshot wounds, therapeutic use of laparoscopy in blunt trauma is not supported by current literature

Operative priorities include:
- rapid control of haemorrhage
  — four-quadrant and pelvic packing
- contamination control
- identification of life-threatening great vessel injuries
- systematic exploration of the entire abdominal cavity
  — addressing injuries as encountered

ABDOMINAL STAB WOUNDS

Background
Stab wounds to the abdomen are infrequently seen compared to the volume of blunt abdominal trauma seen in most emergency departments and trauma centres. Whilst urban American and South African trauma units see a much higher volume of stab wounds than most other places in the western world, all doctors seeing injured patients should be familiar with the evaluation and management of stab wounds.

In busy trauma centres in Australasia, penetrating injury comprises less than 10% of the total trauma volume seen. However, in the subgroup of patients with penetrating abdominal injury, the majority (>80%) are due to stab wounds.

There are important differences between the management of blunt abdominal injury and penetrating abdominal injury, and even between the management of abdominal stab and gunshot wounds.

A stab wound to the abdomen creates challenges in decision-making and management for the doctor attending to the patient. This is especially the case in centres with low volumes of penetrating injury. It is important to understand the following:

- Probabilities of injury
- Value of physical examination
- Investigation options, strengths and weaknesses

- Management options
- Pitfalls

   Timely review by an experienced clinician is an integral and early requirement of care for casualties with penetrating injuries.

Essentials

- Stab wounds are low energy wounds as compared to gunshot wounds and therefore less tissue destruction is caused
- The trajectory of the wounding implement can yield important information about injury probabilities
- Haemodynamic instability mandates early operation
- *Whilst resuscitating a patient is important, control of haemorrhage is paramount (and usually operative)*
- Stable patients with negative abdominal examinations may be managed non-operatively but *only* if being managed by a surgeon with adequate experience and skill in managing penetrating injury
- CT scanning has a limited role in abdominal stab wounds (mainly for the retroperitoneum in back and flank stab wounds)
- FAST is helpful in managing patients with stab wounds near the precordium
- Laparoscopy is a useful way of determining peritoneal penetration in anterior and lateral stab wounds
- Beware of stab wounds in the thoracoabdominal area as there can be injury to structures on *both* sides of the diaphragm and injury to the diaphragm itself (Fig. 2.17)
- All diaphragm injuries require repair

Probabilities of injury/history of Injury

Trajectory information = injury identification
It is likely that the trajectory of the stabbing implement, in combination with its length (if this information is known) and the patient's body habitus, will identify the organs at risk of injury. Below are stab wound locations and organ injury probabilities (in decreasing likelihood for each area). It must, however, be recognized that injury to structures well away from the stab entry wound is common.

- Anterior wounds: omentum, small bowel, colon, stomach and liver. Retroperitoneal structures (major vascular, pancreas and kidney) are less commonly injured
- Lateral wounds: small bowel, colon, spleen, liver, diaphragm, kidney and intrathoracic injury

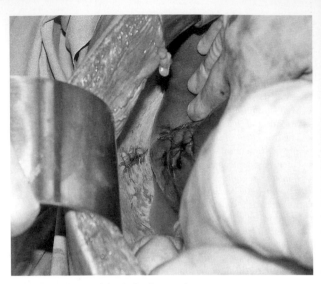

Figure 2.17 Thoracoabdominal stab wound

- Posterior wounds: kidney, pancreas, diaphragm, liver, spleen, duodenum, colon, aorta and inferior vena cava

Clinical examination

The most critical pieces of information are the following:

- Is the patient haemodynamically unstable?
- Does the patient have evidence of peritoneal irritation?
- Is there obvious peritoneal breach?
    — evisceration of omentum, bowel or other intraperitoneal content through the stab wound itself?
- If the answer to any of the above questions is 'yes' then the patient requires a laparotomy
- If the patient is haemodynamically unstable laparotomy must take place immediately
- Remember that a patient's morbidity and mortality rates increase at a continuous rate with ongoing bleeding

 Time is of the essence!

A thorough examination of the patient must be undertaken. The following key points are worth noting.

- Be on the lookout for occult penetrating injuries
  — frequently found on the back, the axillae and groins as well as the perineum
- All stab wounds from the nipple line to the gluteal creases put the intra-abdominal organs at risk of injury
- A digital rectal examination should always be performed

Clinical examination is otherwise of somewhat limited value in the patient with a stab wound to the abdomen. An important exception is that of repeated examinations by a *consistent, experienced* surgeon. This can be helpful in the haemodynamically stable patient with a negative clinical examination and no obvious indication for operative intervention. This can be a management strategy (see sections on Management and Algorithms below) when used appropriately. Physical examination in this setting can be helpful in detecting subtle clinical changes, alerting the surgeon to a patient with significant injury.

Note that physical examination in a patient with altered level of consciousness, regardless of cause (injury, drugs, alcohol, etc.) is often inconsistent and should not be relied upon for decision making.

Investigations
A haemodynamically unstable patient with an abdominal stab wound does not require an investigation—they need an operation!

Bloods
- Blood tests are not of any use in the acute management of a patient with an abdominal stab wound
- The only important tube of blood that must be sent to the laboratory is *the cross-match*

X-rays
- Plain x-rays are neither particularly sensitive nor specific for evidence of intra-abdominal injury
- *Absence of specific signs on x-ray does not equate with absence of injury*
- A plain CXR to assess for haemopneumothorax in stab wounds to the thoracoabdominal region can be helpful
- Radio-opaque markers are always placed over stab wounds to assist with trajectory identification

CT

- *There is no role for CT scanning in the haemodynamically unstable patient*
- *If a patient has an indication for an operation, a CT scan is not required*
- CT is quite sensitive for assessing injury to solid organs but remains limited in its ability to exclude (with adequate confidence) peritoneal penetration and injury to hollow viscus organs or the diaphragm
  — *a negative CT scan cannot be used to exclude injury definitively*
  — CT can be helpful in diagnosing retroperitoneal injury in patients with stab wounds to the back

FAST

- FAST is most useful for assessing stab wounds in which the heart and pericardium are at risk
- It can be used to quickly determine whether a patient has cardiac tamponade or evidence of a pericardial effusion (see Fig. 2.12)
- Absence of pericardial fluid rules out tamponade
- Presence of free fluid within the abdomen indicates peritoneal/pleural penetration and the increased probability of significant injury
- *Absence of free fluid does NOT indicate absence of injury*
  — a negative FAST does not mean the patient has neither peritoneal/pleural penetration nor injury

Diagnostic peritoneal aspiration (DPA) and diagnostic peritoneal lavage

- DPA is simply that part of the test which used to be known as the grossly positive (or negative) DPL
  — aspiration of more than 10 ml of gross blood following insertion of the peritoneal catheter
- DPA is most useful in determining the presence or absence of gross haemoperitoneum
  — in most situations this will clinically be a haemodynamically unstable patient in whom there is some question as to whether a stab wound involves the abdomen or not (i.e. thoracoabdominal wounds) and FAST is unavailable

A haemodynamically unstable patient with a definite abdominal stab wound should go straight to the operating theatre with no delay for any test

- DPL can be helpful in determining the risk of intraperitoneal injury and thus the need for laparotomy
- The threshold values for a positive DPL are lower than for that of blunt injury, with values of greater than 10 000 red blood cells/ml considered positive
  — for amylase and alkaline phosphatase, positive values are those >20 IU

Diagnostic laparoscopy
- Laparoscopy is most useful in determining whether the peritoneum has been breached in penetrating anterior or lateral stab wounds
- 25% of anterior abdominal stab wounds will not penetrate the peritoneal cavity
- Diagnostic laparoscopy is undertaken in *haemodynamically stable* patients to determine whether the peritoneum has been breached
  — in most situations a positive laparoscopy mandates laparotomy to exclude injury
  — adequate inspection of all abdominal organs for evidence of penetrating injury is rarely possible laparoscopically (especially hollow viscus), thereby mandating thorough inspection at laparotomy
- There is no role for laparoscopy in the unstable patient
- Liberal use of laparoscopy in institutions that otherwise mandated laparotomy for stab wounds has significantly decreased the incidence of non-therapeutic laparotomy

Local wound exploration
- Diagnostic laparoscopy has made local exploration of abdominal stab wounds obsolete in many institutions
- Formal exploration of the wound to determine breach of the anterior fascia is occasionally used in stable patients
  — fascial breach mandates laparotomy

Management

<C> ABC
Specific guidelines for the investigation and management of stab wounds to the abdomen are summarized in the algorithms below and in the following specific principles.
- Patients require gastric and urinary decompression with catheters (nasogastric and Foley)
- Patients with ongoing bleeding need an operation, not just 'resuscitation' with colloid and crystalloid

- Haemodynamic instability mandates a rapid transfer to the operating theatre
- In patients requiring early operative intervention for haemorrhage control, excess volumes of i.v. fluid are not given immediately if there is evidence of adequate brain perfusion
  — this will minimize the risk of exacerbating blood loss ('popping the clot') and the resultant 'triad of death' (hypothermia, acidosis and coagulopathy)
- *Do not* poke examining fingers into stab wounds to determine trajectory. This can cause additional injury and worsen bleeding
- Consultant surgeon presence is required early when there is pre-hospital notification of the imminent arrival of a haemodynamically unstable patient with a stab wound to the abdomen
- Decision-making is often time-critical and there is no opportunity to delay important decisions 'until morning,' or some other time considered more convenient, even in the so-called 'stable' patient
- A dying patient with stab wounds in the thoracoabdominal region (below nipple line but above costal margins) needs quick assessment as to whether a laparotomy or thoracotomy is required first
  — chest tubes to assess for haemothorax can be of value

Algorithms
Figures 2.18–2.20 provide general guidelines for the investigation and management of stab wounds to the abdomen.

Pitfalls
- Inaction or delay of critical decision-making
- Inappropriate use of investigations
- Poking fingers into stab wounds to 'see where it goes'
- Delaying involvement of the consultant surgeon
- Managing a patient with stab injuries using similar principles and tactics as for those injured with a blunt mechanism
- Opting for repeat clinical examination as a management strategy when it is either not done as planned or done by someone with minimal experience in managing similar patients
- Mandatory laparotomy for all patients with abdominal stab wounds
- Prioritizing fluid resuscitation when the haemodynamically unstable patient requires urgent surgical therapy
- Doing anything other than operating when the patient has evidence of haemodynamic instability

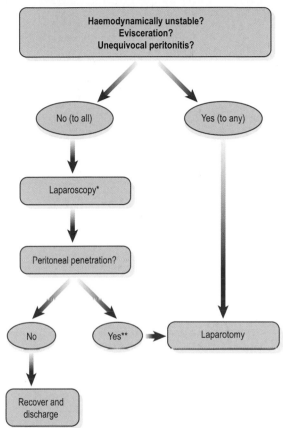

* Laparoscopy is preferred. If adequate resources and surgical experience permit non-operative management, this may be selected. Any evidence of clinical deterioration or development of abdominal signs then mandates laparotomy.

** If penetration is to liver only without ongoing bleeding or diaphragm injury, laparotomy is not required. Patient should be observed closely for at least 48 h before discharge.

Figure 2.18 Algorithm 1. Anterior and lateral stab wounds to the abdomen

FURTHER READING

http://www.trauma.org/abdo/penetrating.html January 2007

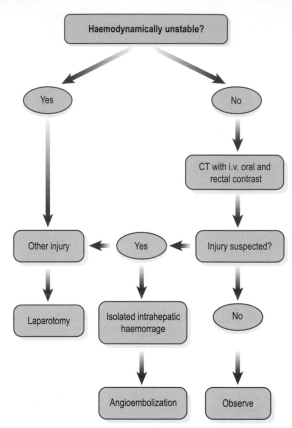

Figure 2.19 Algorithm 2. Posterior stab wounds to the abdomen

---

ABDOMINAL GUNSHOT WOUNDS

Background

The number of firearm assaults has steadily increased in the UK over the past 5 years. Large urban UK emergency departments on average currently manage 10–20 gunshot injuries per year. The increase has occurred despite legislation banning the ownership and use of handguns. Even with this rapid increase, the number of ballistic injuries remains significantly less than that seen in the United States or South Africa. In general, urban shootings tend to

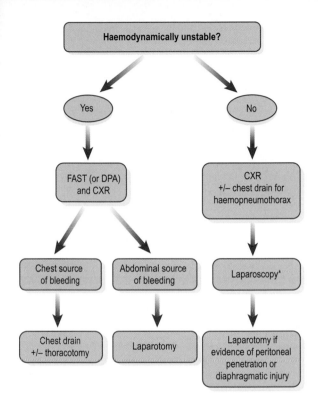

* Beware of pneumoperitoneum for laparoscopy causing tension
pneumothorax in patients with a penetrating wound of the diaphragm

Figure 2.20 Algorithm 3. Thoracoabdominal stab wounds

involve handguns or shotguns and occur in well-known inner city
areas, often being gang- or drug-related. Military grade weapons
are more common in the United States, South Africa and in the
Middle East.

Essentials
- 80–95% of abdominal gunshot wounds will have
  intra-abdominal injuries requiring repair
- Abdominal gunshot wounds most often require *operative
  exploration* and management
- Organ injury depends on the trajectory of the bullet through the
  torso

- The small bowel, colon and liver are the most frequently injured abdominal organs (Table 2.11)
- Multiple perforations of the small bowel are common
- Buttock wounds are associated with a high rate of intra-abdominal injury
- High energy transfer wounds, traditionally from military style weapons, are associated with devastating tissue destruction of solid organs such as the liver (see Section on Ballistics)

Abdominal shotgun wounds

- Shotguns are long guns that fire shells with multiple projectiles. The energy of the shot pellets dissipates rapidly as the target distance increases
- When fired within 5–10 cm of the skin surface, a profound cavitation occurs within the tissues, causing massive destruction

 Treat the wound not the weapon

Resuscitation/immediate management

- Initial resuscitation follows <C>ABC principles (see Section 1 Resuscitation)
- Intra-abdominal bleeding is non-compressible—the priority is getting the patient to the operating room
- Mortality rates increase in haemodynamically abnormal patients with time spent in the resuscitation
- Limit fluid resuscitation to maintain the systolic blood pressure at 90 mmHg or a palpable radial pulse
- Eviscerated bowel
  — cover with sterile saline soaked gauze

TABLE 2.11 Incidence of organ injury following abdominal gunshot wound	
Small bowel	50%
Colon	40%
Liver	30%
Abdominal vascular	25%
Pancreas/duodenum	<10%

Bullets cross surgical boundaries and body cavities

Adjuncts
- Antibiotics should cover Gram-positve and Gram-negative bacteria, and anaerobes
  — e.g. cefuroxime/metronidazole or clindamycin/gentamicin, etc.
- Tetanus prophylaxis
- Foley catheter and nasogastric tube placement in the operating room unless intubated in the trauma bay

Investigation and diagnosis
Clinical evaluation
- A thorough examination is required in all patients with suspected ballistic injury
- The external landmarks defining the abdomen are
  — anterior: nipple level superiorly and inguinal crease inferiorly
  — posterior: tip of scapula superiorly and the buttock crease inferiorly
- *Trajectory* is the key to injury identification
  — however, haemodynamically abnormal patients need surgery not extensive investigation
- Actively hunt for gunshot wounds in 'inaccessible' locations, e.g. axillae or in the buttock folds
- *Remember*:
  — *wounds + bullets = even number*

 Beware of the missing bullet

  — tangential or skive wounds are a diagnosis of exclusion
  — rectal examination for blood

Buttock wounds involve the abdomen until proven otherwise

Place radio-opaque markers on all penetrating wounds

X-ray
- Abdominal x-ray ±lateral with markers over the wounds
  — provides information on location and trajectory of the bullets through the abdomen
- CXR is almost always required to rule out pneumothorax and evaluate for bullet location
- Pelvic x-ray: often the abdominal x-ray does not include the lower pelvis

FAST
Positive FAST

- Signifies significant injury (see Fig.1.10)
- Requires urgent laparotomy
  — a few centres manage selected isolated liver gunshot wounds conservatively
  — this should only be considered in units with significant experience of these injuries

Negative FAST

- *Does not* rule out intra-abdominal injury (sensitivity 50–70%)
- Requires laparotomy or an alternative investigation if the patient is stable and there is probable tangential injury

Blood above and below the diaphragm suggests diaphragm injury.

CT
- *Absolutely contraindicated* in unstable patients and transient responders
- The 'pan-scan' or CT torso topogram
  — provides useful information on the location and trajectory of bullets
  — could replace the abdominal and pelvic x-rays in the haemodynamically *normal* patient
- CT can define trajectory in trauma patients with equivocal physical signs who are *not* haemodynamically abnormal
  — some units consider non-operative approach when *extraperitoneal* tract is away from underlying organs

Laparotomy
- Diagnostic and therapeutic
- No role for laparoscopy

Definitive management

- Laparotomy is always the default (see section on Trauma Laparotomy)

Mandatory laparotomy
Obvious transperitoneal gunshot wounds
Obvious peritoneal signs
Haemodynamically abnormal

- Non-operative management has been described in a few high volume centres
  — isolated liver gunshot wounds
  — trajectory away from the peritoneum on CT
- *Proctoscopy* to rule out extraperitoneal rectal injuries in the evaluation of buttock or transpelvic gunshot wounds
- *Cystography* may be necessary to rule out extraperitoneal bladder injury (see section on Genitourinary Injury)
- Bullets cross boundaries
  — be prepared to extend incisions and operate in other body cavities

 Haemodynamically abnormal patients require urgent exploratory laparotomy

TRAUMA LAPAROTOMY

Indications

- Intra-abdominal bleeding
     gunshot wound
  — haemodynamically unstable from stab wounds and blunt abdominal trauma
- Hollow viscus injury on CT or signs of peritonism
- Penetrating truncal injuries with potential peritoneal injury

Why

- To stop bleeding and prevent exsanguination from vascular/ organ injury
- Control contamination from bowel injury
- Identify and diagnose all organ and hollow viscus injuries

Principles of resuscitation
- <C>ABC
- Fluid, blood and blood product resuscitation
- Operative control of haemorrhage and simultaneous resuscitation
- Consider the need for damage control surgery (see section on Damage Control)
- Remember the operating theatre is a physiologically unfavourable environment for the multiply injured patient
- Broad-spectrum antibiotics preoperatively
- Re-dose antibiotics when large amounts of fluid loss occurs
- Consent not always possible in emergency situation

Principles of surgery

Preparation
- Patient supine ('Crucifix' position with arms out on armboards)
- Ensure anaesthetist is happy with all lines and monitoring
- Prepare rapid fluid infusion equipment
- Position the patient before 'scrubbing up'
- Avoid hypothermia with the placement of warm air convection blankets (Bair Hugger)
- If not already anaesthetized, the patient should be prepped and draped before anaesthesia is induced on the operating table
- Rapidly prep from neck to knees
- Prepare the field with drapes for the worst case scenario
  — have access to both sides of the diaphragm and the groins
  — two large suckers
  — opened large packs
  — consider using cell salvage

Communication
- Talk to the anaesthetist, notify them of plans
- Work as a team with scrub nurse and assistants
- Be aware of your limitations
- Seek senior help sooner rather than later

Aims of surgery
- Restore normal physiology before normal anatomy
- Haemostasis
- Give the anaesthetist time to catch up when bleeding is controlled
- Only perform essential bowel resections
- Close or divert all hollow viscus injuries

Procedure

Access and exposure
- Midline laparotomy incision from below xiphisternum to pubis around umbilicus

Four quadrant packing
- Pack before massive blood loss to control haemorrhage
- Principles of packing
  — pressure stops bleeding
  — pressure vectors in line of tissue planes and capsules (not just random placement)
  — preserve tissue viability
- Avoid 'pack and peek', a dangerous vicious cycle of packing and removal again and again
- After packing remove packs, starting in quadrant with the least amount of bleeding

Exploration
- Explore to determine extent of injury
- Management principles for bleeding include
  — location and control before maintaining flow
  — if there is a major vascular injury consider clamping, temporary intravascular shunting or catheter tamponade before repair
- Actions after bleeding is identified and controlled
  — look for faeces and bile
  — eviscerate small bowel to increase room. 'Run' the bowel twice to look for small bowel injury
- Control and minimize peritoneal contamination by rapid closure of hollow viscus injuries. Use your eyes and your nose!
  — close or divert damaged bowel with tapes, staples or running sutures
  — single resection better than multiple resections
- If stable consider definitive surgery

Closure
- Temporary vs. definitive closure. Temporary abdominal closure used when packs in situ, ACS likely, evidence of bowel oedema, large volumes of blood loss and/or multiple injuries

Documentation and postoperative care
- Ensure accurate operative notes detailing incision, findings, procedure and methods of closure

- Number and location of packs left in situ
- Postoperative plans
- ICU for further physiological optimization
- Postoperative review of patient
- Adequate handover to other surgical teams
- Postoperative immunization in instances of splenectomy

FURTHER READING/COURSES

Definitive Surgical Skills Course (DSTS)
Royal College of Surgeons of England
http://www.rcseng.ac.uk/educational/courses/surgical_trauma.html/
    view?searchterm=trauma January 2007
Definitive Surgical Trauma Course (DSTC)
International Association of Trauma and Surgical Intensive Care (IATSIC)
http://www.iss-sic.ch January 2007

PELVIC TRAUMA

Background

The incidence of pelvic fractures is relatively low, occurring at a
rate of 40/100 000 in the younger population, rising to 500/100 000
in elderly women. However, there is potential for rapid demise of
these patients when haemorrhage is not rapidly controlled.

- Major pelvic trauma is associated with high mortality rates (up
  to 45%)
- Can have complex associated injured patterns
- Patients usually have multisystem injuries
- Many different surgical teams are involved
- Little use of clinical practice guidelines
- If you make a mistake the outcome may be poor

  The spectrum of injury can be quite diverse, ranging from
minor injury to multisystem injury resulting in death. Increasingly
there is a greater understanding of the best way to manage these
patients, particularly those who are haemodynamically unstable.

Classification

There are a number of pelvic fracture classification systems; some
utilize an analysis of force and vectors of energy, while others are
based on radiological and anatomical abnormality. What is crucial
in clinical care is the clinical haemodynamic condition of the
patient as this is what determines outcomes.

- The Young and Burgess classification relates to mechanism of injury and the degree of pelvic disruption. It is divided into
  — anterior compression
  — lateral compression

  It can be further divided into three types (1–3), depending on the amount of bony displacement.

- The Tile classification combines the principles of mechanism of injury and pelvic ring stability

Diagnosis
It is vital to obtain as much pre-hospital information as possible. This should come directly from the scene, providing concise information in the MIST (mechanism, injuries, signs, treatment) format.

Management
- <C>ABC approach with primary, secondary and tertiary surveys
- Damage control in those with critical injuries
  — haemorrhage is the major killer, accounting for 42% of deaths; this occurs in the first 24 h

Over 80% of pelvic injuries are minor and some may not even need admission to hospital. The problem group is that containing the seriously injured patients, who can be identified by the following.

- Mechanism of injury
- Pre-hospital hypotension (BP<90 mmHg)
- Labile BP in resuscitation room
- Base excess >−6
- Elderly patients

Overall mortality rate for pelvic trauma is 16% (range 5–30%); this increases to 27% where there is haemodynamic instability (range 7–42%). Open pelvic fracture is a lethal injury, with a reported mortality rate of 55% (range 50–60)

Physical examination is a sensitive method of determining the presence of a pelvic fracture in a conscious, orientated patient. The presence of pelvic/hip pain or tenderness to palpation over the pelvic girdle or signs of bruising around the pelvic area are an indication to undertake a pelvic x-ray.

- *Pelvic springing should not be done*
- The sensitivity of pelvic springing is only 5% and is painful in the conscious patient

- Don't spring the pelvis but palpate it. There is an important difference between the two

Management (Fig. 2.21)
There are a number of key management questions that need to be resolved in optimizing patient care.

- How do you know if the patient is bleeding?
- Mechanism of injury will provide key information

The four main causes of hypotension in trauma patients are:
- Bleeding
- Haemorrhage
- Haemorrhage
- Exsanguination

- Hypotension suggests that bleeding in a patient with a pelvic fracture is more likely to be from the pelvis (this includes the retroperitoneum) than from the abdomen (60% vs. 30%)
- Rapidly assess each of the major sites of bleeding and exclude them
- The sequence and suggested timelines are shown in Table 2.12

TABLE 2.12 Determining the site of bleeding in the unstable patient		
Site of bleeding	*Diagnosis*	*Time to diagnosis*
External	Visual inspection (look at the patient)	2 min
Long bone fractures	Visual inspection	3 min
Chest	Chest x-ray	10 min
Abdomen	FAST or DPA*	15 min
Pelvis	CT or CTA	45 min
FAST, focused assessment with sonography for trauma; DPA, diagnostic peritoneal lavage; CT, computed tomography; CTA, computed tomography angiography		

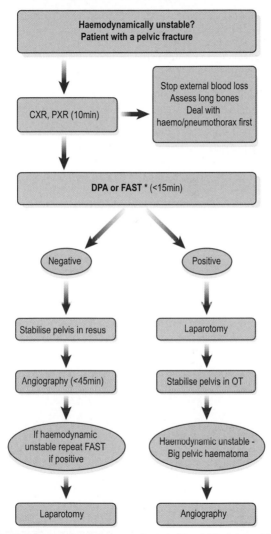

Figure 2.21 Management of a haemodynamically unstable patient with a pelvic fracture. CXR, chest x-ray; PXR, pelvic x-ray; DPA, diagnostic peritoneal aspiration; FAST, focused assessment with sonography in trauma; OT, operating theaters

- Exclude the abdomen as a source of bleeding by investigations
  — there is no role for diagnostic laparotomy in the unstable pelvic trauma patient
- In general the greater the pelvic disruption the greater the risk of bleeding
- An unstable fracture is shown in Figure 2.22 and, after application of a sheet, in Figure 2.23. A vascular blush on CT indicated ongoing bleeding (Fig. 2.24), and immediate embolization was undertaken

Investigations

- FAST (see section on Imaging) is preferable and should be performed as part of the primary survey in unstable patients
- A diagnostic peritoneal aspirate (DPA) is a truncated diagnostic peritoneal lavage and will indicate the presence or absence of blood
  — frank blood on DPA is an indication for immediate laparotomy
  — a common myth is 'that one will get a false positive DPA because of the pelvic fracture'; this is incorrect

How do you stop the bleeding?

The patient who is unstable is potentially bleeding from many different sites. Having cleared the other four potential major sites of haemorrhage (as shown in Table 2.12), the pelvis and

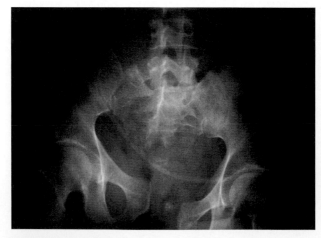

Figure 2.22 An unstable pelvic fracture

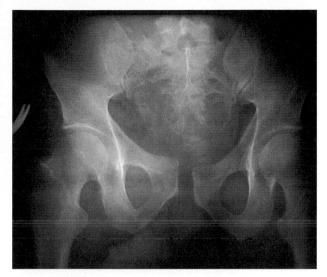

Figure 2.23 Application of a sheet to reduce the pelvis

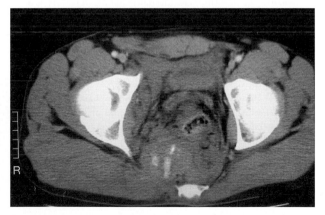

Figure 2.24 A vascular blush on CT indicative of ongoing bleeding

retroperitoneum remain (the fifth site). While venous and bony bleeding are important, it is uncontrolled arterial bleeding that will kill the patient. There are two choices: embolization and surgical ligation of the artery.

- The probability of a pelvic arterial bleed in the hypotensive multisystem trauma patient is $0.80 \times 0.60 = 0.48$
- Of patients in this category going to angiography at least 80% will have active arterial bleeding
- In the hypotensive patient with pelvic fracture, bleeding is from the pelvis in 60%
- Arterial bleeding will be from anterior pelvic arteries in 43% and posterior arteries in 57%, particularly the superior gluteal and lateral sacral

The technique of angioembolization is important, and an initial abdominal flush should be undertaken to give an overall view of potential bleeding sites. Occasionally, unrecognized intra-abdominal bleeding will be identified, usually a mesenteric vascular injury. The patient must be carefully monitored during the procedure.

- The angiography access catheter should be left in place as about 10% will re-bleed

With the advent of 64-slice CT scans there will be increasing opportunities to screen patients for a vascular blush in CT. Currently it is better to go straight to angiography to avoid delays.

- For every 3 min of haemodynamic instability there is a 1% increase in mortality rate
- Time to haemorrhage control remains a key to good outcome

When and how should you fix the pelvis?
The patient should have a pelvic sling or binder such as the TPOD™ (Figure 2.25) applied in the resuscitation room when there is a pelvic diathesis. The knees or ankles should be gently tied together to approximate the pelvis further.

- The patient should *not* have an external fixator applied before haemorrhage control in the pelvis has been achieved
   — an external fixator is not ideal as it does not stop arterial bleeding, it is cumbersome and it is a potential source of wound infection in the skin

The urinary catheter?
A urinary catheter should be passed in all cases *except*

- where there is blood at the meatus
- a high riding prostate

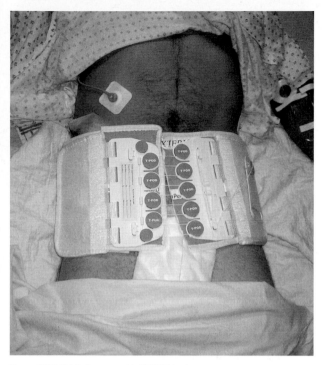

Figure 2.25 Pelvic fracture with TPOD™ in situ

There should be only one attempt at catheterization. If this is unsuccessful, a retrograde urethogram should be performed.

COMPOUND PELVIC INJURIES

These pose a specific challenge related in part to the extra force and injury sustained by the patient. There is a much greater chance of rapid exsanguination which can be venous as well as arterial in this small subset of patients. Rapid transfer to the operating theatre is preferable in this group. There is often obvious indication for surgery, usually for either haemorrhage control or colostomy.

There is no need for abdominal investigations. The patient should be taken straight to the operating room for a laparotomy and damage control abdominal procedures

FURTHER READING

Burgess A R, Tile M 1991 Fractures of the pelvis. In: Rockwood C, Green D (eds) Fractures in adults. JB Lippincott, Philadelphia, p 1399–1442

Heetveld M J, Harris I, Schlaphoff G, Sugrue M 2004 Guidelines for the management of haemodynamically unstable pelvic fracture patients. Australia and New Zealand Journal of Surgery 74:520–529

The Eastern Association for the Surgery of Trauma website http://www.east.org/tpg/pelvis.pdf 1 October 2005

Tile M 1988 Pelvic ring fractures: should they be fixed? Journal of Bone and Joint Surgery (Br) 70:1–12

GENITOURINARY INJURY

Background

Approximately 10% of trauma patients will have a urological injury. It is important to consider the genitourinary (GU) system during the initial evaluation as suspicion is the key to diagnosis. While haematuria is often the initial sign of urological trauma, substantial injuries can exist in the absence of red blood cells.

Initial evaluation

- A detailed history of the traumatic event can help guide the initial evaluation and raise the suspicion of possible urological injury
- The presence of blood at the urethral meatus implies injury to the urethra and mandates evaluation with a retrograde urethrogram (RUG) *prior* to attempts at Foley urinary catheter placement
- Urinalysis of the initial aliquot of urine is important as haematuria can clear quickly
- Haematuria can result from injury anywhere along the GU tract — multiple concomitant urological injuries are possible
- Penetrating injuries of the chest, abdomen, flanks or pelvis can result in significant GU injury

There is no relationship between the degree of haematuria and the severity of injury

RENAL TRAUMA

Approximately 80% of renal injuries are the result of blunt trauma and 20% result from penetrating trauma.

> Absence of haematuria can exist in the setting of major injuries to the renal pedicle or pelvic–ureteral junction

Diagnosis

Appropriate imaging allows diagnosis and classification of GU injuries, and determines the need for and appropriate timing of operative management. The following patients should be investigated.

- Patients with penetrating trauma and any degree of haematuria who are haemodynamically stable
- Patients with blunt trauma and
  — gross haematuria
  — microhaematuria and systolic blood pressure <90 mmHg at any point since injury
- Any mechanism of injury suggesting possible renal trauma, especially
  — high speed deceleration injuries (fall from height, high speed motor vehicle collision)
  — penetrating trauma near the renal tract

Investigations

- Assess injury to the GU tract and associated organs
- Assess function of contralateral side to help in planning further care
- Diagnose pre-existing GU conditions which may contribute to the injury or its management

CT with intravenous contrast

- Current imaging modality of choice
- Initial scan following contrast administration should be followed by a delayed scan 10–20 min later to evaluate for extravasation of urine and/or collecting system injury

CT cystogram

- Initial CT scan is followed by a CT cystogram with distension of the bladder with 300 ml of dilute contrast
- Evaluate for intraperitoneal and extraperitoneal bladder injury

IVU
- Second-line imaging choice
- Must include nephrotomograms and full evaluation of bilateral kidneys with contrast excretion into ureters to be a complete study

Intraoperative one-shot IVU
- Useful in haemodynamically unstable patients taken directly to theatre for laparotomy prior to radiological investigations
- Allows assessment of major renal injuries, contrast extravasation and function of contralateral side

> **How to perform one shot intravenous urogram**
> - 2 ml contrast per kilogram (or 150 ml contrast) given as an i.v. bolus
> - Single shot flat plate plain film 10 min later

Angiography
- Useful in the patient with suspected renal arterial thrombosis or segmental renal arterial injuries
- Therapeutic interventions may be carried out concurrently
  — e.g. stenting, embolization of bleeding vessels

Management

The American Association for the Surgery of Trauma (AAST) organ injury scale for renal injuries can be used to guide management. These are available at http://www.aast.org/injury/injury.html (accessed 1 June 2006)

- Stable patients with AAST grade I–III injuries and non-vascular grade IV injuries can safely be managed non-operatively
- Operative exploration is indicated in
  — unstable patients with persistent haemorrhage believed to be caused by renal injury
  — patients with a renal hilar or pedicle injury (grade V)
  — patients with pulsatile or expanding haematomas

> Patients with suspected urological injury explored *prior* to complete imaging should have a one-shot IVU

- Nephrectomy should be performed when renal injuries are considered unreconstructable or when patients are clinically unstable from other injuries

Complications of renal injury
- Urinoma/haematoma
- Perinephric abscess formation
- Hypertension
- Hydronephrosis
- Renal insufficiency
- Delayed haemorrhage—can occur between 2 and 36 days

URETERIC INJURY

Ureteric injuries from trauma are rare and lack specific associated signs. A high index of suspicion must be maintained to diagnose such injuries early, and so prevent late and significant complications.

- The majority result from penetrating trauma
  — gunshot wounds > stab wounds
- Blunt injury is rare
- Frequently occur in conjunction with multiple associated injuries
- *Haematuria is NOT a consistent finding and its absence does NOT rule out injury*
- Higher complication rates are likely if the injury is recognized late

Children with rapid deceleration injuries may experience hyperextension and resultant pelviureteric junction disruption

Diagnosis and investigations
- Maintain a high index of suspicion
- CT scan with i.v. contrast and delayed excretory views
  — first choice imaging study in stable patients
  — extravasation of contrast is diagnostic
- IVU
  — second choice study
  — One-shot IVU is generally not sufficient
- Retrograde pyelogram
  — very specific but sometimes difficult to perform in the setting of multiple concomitant injuries and/or active resuscitation
- Intraoperative exploration of penetrating injuries involving the retroperitoneum and/or evaluation of retroperitoneal haematomas is very accurate

- Intraoperative injection of indigo carmine either intravenously or directly into the renal pelvis can demonstrate extravasation and guide exploration

Management

Keys to successful repair include

- Adequate debridement of devitalized tissue
- Proximal and distal mobilization allowing for a tension-free anastomosis
- Proximal and distal spatulation
- Repair over a ureteric stent
- Adequate postoperative retroperitoneal drainage

Unstable or coagulopathic patients may be best managed with formation of a cutaneous ureterostomy or ureteral ligation and nephrostomy tube placement.

Complications

- Urine leak can be managed with percutaneous nephrostomy tube placement ± antegrade stent placement
- Urinoma formation indicates the need for percutaneous drainage

BLADDER INJURIES

Bladder injuries represent a small portion of urological trauma which are generally easily diagnosed and repaired. With timely and appropriate management, complications are rare.

- The majority result from blunt trauma
  — motor vehicle collisions/falls
- 95% of bladder injuries are associated with gross haematuria
- Highly associated with pelvic fracture

Diagnosis and investigations

- Plain film or CT cystogram (Table 2.13)
- Excretion phase of CT/IVU is *not* sufficient; there is a high rate of false negative results
- If *no* blood is present at the meatus and digital rectal examination is normal, gentle urethral catheterization may be attempted

Maintain a low threshold for performing retrograde urethrogram, especially with pelvic trauma

TABLE 2.13 Comparison of CT cystogram with plain film cystogram	
CT cystogram	Plain film cystogram
Requires two scans: — early filling scan after gravity installation of 100 cm³ contrast — complete fill scan after gravity instillation of 350 cm³ contrast	Multiple images required: — scout film — anteroposterior films with full bladder after gravity instillation of 350 cm³ 30% dilute contrast — anteroposterior films after drainage

Bladder injury classifications/management

- Contusion—injury to bladder without obvious perforation
    - Managed conservatively with or without a Foley catheter
    - Patients with pelvic haematomas may require a Foley until haematoma resolves
- Intraperitoneal rupture: usually a blow-out injury at dome
    - contrast may outline loops of bowel or track along lateral gutters
    - requires operative repair
- Extraperitoneal rupture: 'flame shaped' extravasation into perivesical tissue
    - can generally be managed non-operatively with Foley catheter
    - repeat cystogram at 10 days to confirm healing
- Penetrating injuries to the bladder should be explored operatively and repaired

It is important to evaluate the distal ureters for concurrent injury

Contraindications to *non-operative* management of extraperitoneal bladder ruptures

- Patients undergoing laparotomy for non-urological injuries
- Urinary tract infection
- Inadequate bladder drainage via urethral Foley
- Presence of bone fragments in bladder
- Patients undergoing internal fixation of pelvic injuries (high infectious precautions)

Disruption of a pelvic haematoma may result in significant bleeding

Complications
- Urinoma/abscess formation
- Incontinence
- Fistula
- Stricture
- Neurogenic injury

URETHRAL INJURY

The vast majority of urethral injuries occur in men and are the result of blunt trauma. Rarely, women sustain urethral injuries, usually associated with pelvic fractures. Male urethral injuries are classically divided by location.

- Anterior urethral injuries
  — typically caused by straddle injuries or perineal trauma
  — crushing of bulbar urethra against pubic ramus results in contusion or laceration
  — RUG demonstrates extravasation below urogential diaphragm
- Posterior urethral injuries
  — 5 to 10% association with pelvic fractures, 15% with concurrent bladder injury
  — highly associated with significant co-morbidities from pelvic bleeding
  — result from shearing of membranous urethra

Diagnosis
- The mainstay of diagnosis is the RUG
- Patients presenting with any of the following should have a RUG
  — blood at the urethral meatus
  — a high riding prostate (difficult to palpate)
  — acute inability to urinate
  — penile/perineal contusion
  — a mechanism of injury consistent with urethral injuries
- Patients transferred or arriving with a catheter in place and suspicion of urethral injury should undergo either a pericatheter urethrogram or a voiding cystourethrogram (VCUG) to evaluate for injury

Management
Treatment is controversial as these injuries are relatively rare and are usually associated with significant concurrent injuries.

Retrograde urogram
- Place the patient in 30° oblique position
- Place Foley catheter in fossa navicularis and fill balloon with 2–3 cm^3
- Stretch penis to straighten anterior urethra
- Slowly inject undiluted contrast and take plain film images at 10 cm^3 intervals

- The focus should be on establishing urinary drainage and managing life-threatening injuries

Anterior injuries
- Partial disruption may be managed with urethral Foley placement
- Endoscopic placement of Foley catheter to stent urethra may be useful in some cases
- Typically treated with placement of suprapubic catheter followed by evaluation with VCUG at 3–4 weeks
- Open repair and urethroplasty generally delayed for at least 3 months

Posterior injuries
- Immediate open repair is associated with high rates of incontinence, impotence and stricture
- In haemodynamically stable patients with limited associated injuries, primary endoscopic realignment may be attempted
  — when successful, this approach may lower the rate of stricture; however, there is potential for significant morbidity
- Typically, posterior injuries are managed with the placement of a suprapubic tube to allow urinary diversion, followed by definitive repair in 3–6 months
- Open suprapubic catheter placement is preferred to allow for placement of large calibre tube
- Concurrent bladder injuries should be primarily repaired

Complications
- Stricture
- Erectile dysfunction
- Incontinence

SCROTAL INJURY

Due to its external and dependent location, the scrotum is
vulnerable to trauma. Injuries can involve any of the scrotal
contents, with 85% of injuries being blunt.

 Beware of traumatic testicular torsion

- Examination can be difficult secondary to swelling and pain
- Occasionally large scrotal swelling may result from pelvic
  haematoma with extravasation
- The goal is to establish the extent of injury and the need for
  operative intervention

Investigation

- Scrotal ultrasound is the single best imaging study for
  determining injury; however, its success is user-dependent
  — need to establish location, integrity and preserved vascular
    flow to both testicles
- Indications for scrotal exploration following blunt scrotal
  trauma include
  — testicular rupture
  — testicular torsion
  — presence of large haematocoele
  — testicular dislocation
- Except for superficial scrotal skin injuries, all penetrating injuries
  warrant surgical exploration
- Equivocal findings on scrotal ultrasound should prompt surgical
  exploration

PENILE INJURY

- May be penetrating or blunt
- Extent of injury can frequently be determined by physical
  examination
  — if Buck's fascia is intact, the haematoma will be confined to
    the penis
  — if Buck's fascia is torn, the haematoma will spread along
    Colle's fascia and Scarpa's fascia onto the perineum and
    abdominal wall

- Penetrating injuries to the penis require surgical exploration and definitive repair
- Blunt penile fracture is a rupture of the tunica albuginea surrounding the corpora cavernosa
  — injury occurs almost exclusively to the erect penis when excessive angulation force is applied
- Associated urethral injury in 10–20%
  — perform RUG as necessary
- Management with immediate operative exploration and repair of tunica reduces early and late complications, including penile abscess and fibrosis and penile curvature

EXTREMITY TRAUMA

ORTHOPAEDIC INJURY

Background

Musculoskeletal injury is very common in major trauma. The incidence of significant orthopaedic injury in severely injured patients is 78%. The vast majority of permanent disability after major trauma is a result of musculoskeletal or CNS injury. In major trauma, orthopaedic injury occurs as part of the following scenarios.

- Multiple orthopaedic injuries only
- Multisystem trauma, with multiple orthopaedic injuries
- Multisystem injury with minor (not life-threatening) orthopaedic injury

RESUSCITATION

Orthopaedic haemorrhage control

- Address and control sources of catastrophic haemorrhage
- Direct pressure controls most peripheral bleeding
- Broken bones bleed
  — femur 1000 cm^3
  — tibia 750 cm^3
  — pelvic fracture ±2000 cm^3
- Splinting reduces blood loss and should be applied early (pre-hospital ideally)
- Continued hypotension is *unlikely* to be due to an isolated long bone fracture
  — look elsewhere

- Pelvic bleeding kills
  — unstable pelvic fractures need to be stabilized quickly
  — see section on Pelvic Fracture

20–25% of all major trauma deaths have a pelvic fracture

Secondary survey
Orthopaedic injuries are usually identified during the secondary survey.

History—mechanism of injury
- A detailed history is essential (from patient, witnesses, paramedics and police)
- Patterns of orthopaedic injury exist
  — e.g. falls from a height can result in calcaneal fractures, tibial plateau fractures and spinal fractures
  — see section on Mechanism of Injury
- It is important to be aware of these patterns and look carefully for associated injuries

Examination
- Major long bone fractures are usually obvious
  — limb often deformed/short
- Up to 10% of 'lesser' fractures may be missed during the initial resuscitation phase (see section on Tertiary Survey)

 All fractures are important to the patient

- Assess major joints for active and passive range of movement and stability
- Carefully palpate long bones (arm/forearm/thigh/calf) for
  — pain, crepitus, abnormal movement
- Look carefully for open fractures
  — open fractures are an orthopaedic emergency and must not be missed
  — there may only be a puncture wound
  — a wound associated with a fracture often bleeds with local pressure
  — photograph wound
  — cover loosely in aqueous povidone iodine-soaked gauze and loose crepe bandage/cling film

—   do not remove the dressing until the patient is in theatre
    (within 6 h)
—   give i.v. broad-spectrum antibiotic *as per local protocol* (local
    protocols often exist)
—   administer tetanus toxoid/immunoglobulin
• Don't forget to logroll and assess all of the spine
• Splint the injury site
  —   splinting a fracture reduces pain, reduces further damage to
      local structures and reduces blood loss
  —   splint the joint above and below the fracture site
  —   check distal neurological status and circulation before and
      after applying splint
  —   femoral fractures are placed in a traction splint
      e.g. Thomas splint, pneumatic splint
  —   other lower limb fractures are put in plaster of Paris
      back-slabs or vacuum splints
  —   upper limb fractures are placed in broad arm slings, collar
      and cuff or plaster of Paris back-slabs as appropriate

> Do not defer splint placement because the patient is going to
> theatre immediately
>   In major trauma delays are frequent and the splint is easily
> forgotten

Radiological imaging

• Have a low threshold for obtaining radiographs of areas of
  concern
  —   patients are often distracted with other injuries, and bruising
      and swelling is not always apparent early
• If radiographs are poor quality, they need to be repeated and *not*
  forgotten about
• The best time and place for plain radiographs is usually the
  emergency department (as long as the patient's general condition
  is acceptable)

Radiological imaging—specialized imaging

• CT, MRI and contrast studies are performed according to
  specific requirements and the patient's general condition

Injury recognition: high energy limb injuries

• In any injury, the extent of the injury sustained is proportional
  to the amount of energy absorbed by the tissues at the time of
  the injury

- It is important to be able to recognize high energy limb injuries
  — the surgical fracture and soft tissue management is complex and therefore the prognosis and outcome is correspondingly worse

History
- Any road traffic accident, driver, passenger or pedestrian
- Falls from a height
- An injury associated with general or localized crushing
- Missile wounds
- Contamination from the scene of the accident
- A history of entrapment for any period
- A history of limb ischaemia

Examination
- Large or multiple wounds
- Imprints or contamination from dirt or tyres
- Crush or burst wounds
- Skin degloving
  — skin is intact but devascularized owing to shear between the deep fascia and subcutaneous tissues
- More than one fracture in the same limb
- Evidence of associated compartment syndrome
- Evidence of associated vascular injury
- Evidence of associated nerve injury

Plain radiography
- Segmental fractures
  — fracture at more than one level in same bone
- Highly comminuted fractures
- Wide displacement of bone fragments
- Evidence of air in the soft tissues

Timing of surgery

 Patients with major trauma are not too sick for surgery—they are too sick to delay surgery

Patients with major trauma and multiple injuries have altered physiology because of the injuries sustained. An injury of any description results in an inflammatory reaction which is proportional to the size of the injury. The inflammatory reaction is designed to promote healing and repair, but it can become prolonged or exaggerated, leading to systemic inflammatory response syndrome, acute respiratory distress syndrome (ARDS) etc.

The aim of all treatment is to control the inflammatory reaction and restore normal physiology and homeostasis as soon as possible. Orthopaedic surgery can increase or decrease this inflammatory response and systemic physiology.

Reducing the overall inflammatory response
- Remove necrotic/devitalized tissue by debridement/fasciotomy
- Reduce blood loss by splinting/stabilizing fractures
- Reduce pain by splinting/stabilizing fractures
- Reduce ischaemia by joint relocation/fasciotomy/stabilizing fractures

Increasing the overall inflammatory response
- Excessive surgery—blood loss/hypothermia

> Orthopaedic intervention must be beneficial and not harmful to the patient

Orthopaedic intervention
- Life-saving thoracic, abdominal, pelvic and neurosurgical procedures are undertaken first
- If the patient's condition is suitable proceed to limb-saving procedures
- Communication and coordination with colleagues in other specialties is essential
- In critically ill patients, optimal fracture care can be suboptimal acute trauma care
- The initial goal is patient survival
- Long-term musculoskeletal function is of less immediate concern
- Adhere to general orthopaedic principles
- Optimal individual fracture fixation techniques need to be modified to treat overall orthopaedic injuries
- Procedures undertaken in stepwise fashion
- Patient's physiology assessed at each stage before advancing to the next stage

Danger signs
- Hypoxia
- Hypothermia
- Abnormal clotting
- Acidosis
- Increased intracranial pressure

Sometimes trauma patients need the ICU more than additional surgical exposure

ORTHOPAEDIC SURGICAL PRIORITIES

Ischaemia correction
- Identify and correct the source of haemorrhagic shock
- Reduce dislocated joints
- Splint limbs in anatomical position
- Stabilize fractures if associated vascular repair is required
- Fasciotomy for compartment syndrome
- Avoid hypothermia

Wound care
- Open fractures are an orthopaedic emergency and need to be debrided and stabilized within 6 h
- A tourniquet is placed on the limb but is not inflated unless *absolutely necessary*
- Remove contaminants
- Excise necrotic or devitalized tissue and skin margins
- Wounds are extended to achieve adequate exposure of soft tissues and bone ends
- Longitudinal wound extension is safest but seek plastic surgical advice if available as potential reconstructive options may need to be considered
- Open fractures need copious irrigation/debridement
  — minimum 6 l warm saline
  — pressurized 'pulse' lavage aids removal of debris, but may force debris deeper into tissues
- Viability of muscle is assessed according to the 4 "c's"
  — colour, contractility, consistency, capacity to bleed
- *Do not close wounds primarily*
  — it is permissible to close the surgically extended portion of wound *only*

- A joint capsule may be closed, leaving the skin open
- If possible, bone ends should be covered in viable soft tissue
  — without compromising surrounding tissues
- Bone fragments without healthy soft-tissue attachments (blood supply) are removed
- The wound is covered in povidone iodine-soaked gauze and bandaged loosely
- All wounds need to be re-inspected within 48 h
- This is usually performed in theatre with general anaesthetic and a plastic surgeon if required
- Definitive wound closure (plastic surgery) should be within 5 days of the injury
- Use of antibiotics until definitive wound closure is controversial

> Intravenous antibiotics are not an alternative to debridement, dead tissue is not perfused

- After *wound care* the fracture must be *stabilized*
- The choice of stabilization depends on
  — fracture configuration
  — fracture grade
  — extent of soft-tissue damage/contamination
  — surgical experience
- External fixation or intramedullary nail is used for diaphyseal fractures
- Plating or external fixation is undertaken for proximal or distal metaphyscal fractures

Open fracture classification (Gustilo and Anderson)
I   Low energy fracture pattern wound <1 cm
II Low energy fracture pattern wound >1 cm
III High energy fracture pattern
    A Adequate soft tissue coverage
    B Soft tissue reconstruction required
    C Associated nerve or vascular injury requiring repair

Long bone stabilization

- Femoral shaft fractures and pelvic stabilization should be undertaken during initial general anaesthetic if the patient's general condition allows

- Patients benefit from early stabilization of long bone fractures (within 24 h)
  — reduces overall patient morbidity and mortality (controversial)
  — excellent pain control
  — avoids traction and associated difficulty sitting and moving around the bed, with potential respiratory system benefits
- Femoral shaft fractures are the next priority after pelvic stabilization
  — closed intramedullary nailing is the treatment of choice for femoral fractures
  — infection rate ~1%
  — non-union rate ~1%
- If this is not possible owing to the patient's general condition, a temporary external fixator should be applied
- After femoral stabilization, proceed to stabilization of other long bones if the patient's condition permits

> If the patient has significant associated injuries, the timing of stabilization has to be weighed against ongoing systemic instability
> It can be deferred until operative exposure is less of a risk if necessary

Other fractures
- Pelvic fractures and femoral fractures should be stabilized under initial general anaesthesia if the patient's physiology permits
- Femoral neck fractures and talar neck fractures are the next priority to reduce the risk of avascular necrosis in major weightbearing joints
- This is followed by repair of
  — metaphyseal distal femoral fracture
  — proximal and distal metaphyseal tibial fractures
  — ankle fractures
  — foot fractures
  — wrist/elbow fractures
- The progressive stabilization of 'other fractures' depends on numerous factors
  — the patient's general condition
  — requirement for specialized imaging
    complex intra-articular fractures often need CT scans prior to reconstruction

— soft tissue swelling is common, especially in foot and ankle fractures

  it may take 2 weeks to settle enough for internal fixation to be considered

  a temporary 'bridging' external fixator can be used as temporary skeletal stabilization

— if there are combined upper and lower limb fractures, consider stabilizing upper limb fractures early to allow shared weightbearing

— surgical and nursing expertise

— implant availability

— fatigue of theatre staff

Reaming for femoral shaft fracture—reaming and pulmonary failure

- Reaming involves removing the intramedullary contents of a long bone and creating an appropriate passage to allow insertion of a nail

- The process results in the release of some of the medullary contents into the circulation

- There is concern that using reamed femoral intramedullary (cannulated) nails in presence of blunt chest trauma can lead to ARDS

- The evidence is mainly experimental and often based on animal studies and intact femora

- It is possible that inserting femoral nails (smaller diameter, solid nails) without reaming the intramedullary canal is safer

- It is probably sensible to limit reaming and use smaller solid (not cannulated) intramedullary femoral nails in patients with severe chest trauma

Unreamed, smaller diameter, solid nails may have an increased risk of implant failure and non-union

Femoral nailing has significant benefits on patients with major trauma, and delay in stabilization can be detrimental to patients' physiology

Principles of external fixation

- System of skeletal stabilization using percutaneous pins and connecting rods remote from site of injury

- It is suitable for many different injury patterns
- Often used for provisional stabilization in the multiple trauma setting, but can also be used for definitive stabilization in certain circumstances
- Relatively quick and easy
- Bloodless
- Easily adjustable interoperatively and postoperatively
- Image intensifier useful but not essential
- Can be an alternative to intramedullary nailing if patient's general condition dictates
- Two half pins above and below fracture site are adequate for provisional stabilization of diaphyseal fractures
- Pin insertion into subcutaneous border of bone (tibia, pelvis, ulna) minimizes risk of neurovascular injury
- In the humerus and femur, pins are inserted adjacent to the lateral intermuscular septum (safe zone)
- If used as a provisional method of stabilization, it must be converted to an intramedullary nail within 2 weeks to minimize the risk of long-term osteomyelitis occurring as a result of pin tract bacterial contamination of the medullary canal
- In complex articular fractures the joint can be 'bridged' with the pins inserted above and below the involved joint
  — maintains joint reduction and fracture alignment by ligamentotaxis

Compartment syndrome

- Increased pressure of soft tissues in an enclosed compartment of the extremity
  — leads to ischaemia and necrosis of the soft tissues in the compartment, resulting in fibrosis and nerve damage
- Occurs most commonly in fractures of the lower leg, forearm and foot, and in patients with major trauma
- Usually occurs with fractures but can occur with crush injury or contusion
- Easy to miss if patient is being resuscitated, or is paralysed or intoxicated
- Signs of compartment syndrome
  — pain: more than expected, unrelieved by opiates
  — pain unrelieved by immobilization of the fractured limb
  — never assume pain is from the bone
  — pain on passive stretching of the affected compartment
  — a tense, swollen limb

> Pulselessness, pallor, paraesthesia and paralysis are *late* signs, manifesting after the damage has occurred

- Compartment pressures can be measured using an isolated reading or continuous monitoring
- Normal pressure in muscle compartment is 0 mmHg
- Compartment syndrome is present when differential pressure between *diastolic* blood pressure and compartment pressure is less than 30 mmHg, or if the absolute pressure in the compartment is more than 40 mmHg
- Care with prolonged hypotension, poor peripheral perfusion (when diastolic blood pressure is already low)

Treatment
Treatment is by fasciotomy.
- Fasciotomy should be performed if there is an obvious diagnosis or if there is any concern about the diagnosis
- Unnecessary fasciotomy is preferable to compartment syndrome
- Release all dressings and splints down to the skin
  — blood-encrusted bandages act as tourniquets
- Release all compartments in the zone of injury
  — skin and fascia incised
  — cosmetic outcome should not be a concern
    Look again at 48 h (under general anaesthesia), when the decision to close fasciotomy wound or skin graft is taken

 Compartment syndrome can occur in open fractures

Limb salvage versus amputation
- Difficult decision unless the limb is not viable or reconstruction is obviously going to result in a non-functional limb
- Senior decision, consultation with colleagues is recommended
- Need to discuss options with patient preoperatively if possibility of amputation
- Photographic evidence useful
- Detailed notes regarding decision-making process are essential
- MESS score (see section on Scoring Systems) is a useful guide for decision-making but *not absolute*

- Other factors involved in decision-making include
  - extent of bony injury
  - nerve supply; protective sensation is critical to good outcome especially posterior tibial nerve in lower limb trauma; damage leaves the sole of the foot insensate
  - crush injuries do relatively badly
- Lower limb vs. upper limb as prostheses are significantly more functional in the lower limb
- Physiological reserve: comorbidity (diabetes, cardiovascular and respiratory status) before injury
- Smoking
- Economic, psychological and social factors
- Mass casualty situation—resource implications

 Attempted limb salvage can result in increased sepsis, cost and psychosocial morbidity

PERIPHERAL VASCULAR INJURY

Recognition
Clinically significant peripheral arterial injury is identified by the presence of one or more *hard* signs.

Hard signs of arterial injury
- Pulsatile bleeding
- Expanding haematoma
- Absent palpable distal pulses
- Cold, pale limb
- Palpable thrill
- Audible bruit

 The presence of a hard sign mandates further investigation and treatment

Historically, soft signs of vascular injury have been used to indicate the need for vascular imaging.

> **Soft signs of vascular injury**
> - Peripheral nerve deficit
> - History of haemorrhage at scene
> - A reduced but palpable pulse
> - An injury in proximity to a major artery

However, there is good long-term evidence to show that in the absence of a hard sign of arterial injury there will be no clinically significant vascular injury.

Diagnostic adjuncts
- The role of handheld Doppler ultrasound in the assessment of peripheral vascular injury is contentious
- Many institutions continue to assess for a peripheral pulse using Doppler and use an ankle–brachial pressure of 0.9 as a cut-off below which further investigation is required

However:

- If a pulse is palpable, the injury is not clinically relevant and the limb can safely be observed
- If a pulse is not palpable, there is a clinically relevant injury regardless of the presence or absence of a Doppler signal

Duplex ultrasound has not yet found a place in the evaluation of vascular trauma.

Angiography
Angiography is the gold standard for investigation of vascular injury. However, it is unnecessary in the majority of peripheral vascular injuries as the site of injury is usually known. Exceptions to this are

- Multiple level injuries
- Shotgun wounds
- Blunt trauma

Angiography, if necessary, is best performed on the operating table. Transfer to the angiography suite should be reserved for haemodynamically stable patients with torso injuries.

Immediate management

<C> Catastrophic haemorrhage
See section on <C> catastrophic haemorrhage.

On-table angiogram technique
1. Ensure the patient is on an x-ray table
2. Insert an angiography sheath into a proximal vessel (common femoral) using a puncture needle and Seldinger technique
3. Attach an extension set and three-way tap to the sheath.
4. Inject 20–40 ml of contrast i.v. under fluoroscopic visualization
5. If using plain radiographs, begin injecting contrast at a rapid pace. From the start of injecting, the delay to take the x-ray in seconds is half the distance from catheter to injury in centimetres
6. Flush the catheter with heparinized saline

- Direct finger pressure
  - apply direct pressure to the bleeding point if it is obvious
  - otherwise apply pressure over a major artery at a bony prominence proximal to the level of the injury
    over the common femoral artery at the femoral head
    over the brachial artery at the elbow
    over the axillary artery in the axilla
  - assign one person to this task
    do not rely on gauze or bandages to provide adequate compression
- *Minimal* volume resuscitation is indicated prior to haemorrhage control
- Transfer immediately to the operating room
- Gain proximal and distal control of the injury
- Decide on damage control procedure or definitive repair based on the patient's physiology
- *Damage control*
  - vascular shunt
  - ligation
- *Definitive repair*
  - simple repair
  - vein or graft interposition
  - ligation and bypass
- Consider fasciotomy in all patients but especially in those with
  - episodes of hypotension
  - prolonged ischaemic time (>4 h)
  - concurrent venous injury
  - blast injuries

Ischaemic limb

- Gain intravenous access
- Transfer immediately to the operating room
- In the absence of major active haemorrhage elsewhere, volume resuscitate as necessary
- On-table angiography if indicated
- Gain proximal and distal control
- Consider fasciotomy
  — if performing a fasciotomy, insert a shunt into damaged vessels to restore flow first
- Repair vessel(s) using direct repair, graft interposition or ligation and bypass as indicated
- If venous repair is possible, repair the vein prior to the artery

Special situations

Arterial injury associated with long bone fracture A decision should be made whether to stabilize the fracture or restore blood flow first.

- If an external fixator can be placed rapidly, this should be performed first
- If orthopaedic repair will take longer than 20–30 min, or if the ischaemia time is already prolonged:
  — *the vascular injury should be assessed first and flow restored before long bone fixation*

The damaged vessels should be rapidly accessed and flow restored with a temporary shunt. The long bone fixation should be performed and, finally, definitive vascular repair. This allows repair with the fracture reduced and with the limb at normal length, and avoids disruption of the repair during orthopaedic fixation.

Dislocated knee

- If there is no palpable pulse there is an arterial injury that requires repair
- Angiography is not indicated as the level of injury is known
- The patient should be transferred to the operating room for popliteal artery exploration and repair

Tibial fractures with vascular compromise

- Angiography will show severe pruning or narrowing of the crural vessels
- Wide four-compartment fasciotomy should be performed
- Crural vessel reconstruction is not indicated
  — if all three vessels are completely disrupted, the limb is inevitably not salvageable

Compartment syndrome

Compartment syndrome is likely with

- Episodes of hypotension
- Prolonged ischaemic time (>4 h)
- Concurrent venous injury
- Blast injuries
- Vasoconstrictor use (typically cocaine)

Patients with any of these factors should be considered to be at high risk for compartment syndrome and prophylactic fasciotomy considered.

If patients are being observed, persistent severe pain in the limb which is worse on passive extension of the affected muscle group, is the primary sign of the presence of a compartment syndrome.

 Distal pulses are present until the late stages of compartment syndrome

Examination is impossible if the patient is unconscious, has a spinal cord injury or is receiving epidural anaesthesia. In these situations clinical examination, feeling for 'tense compartments' is *totally unreliable*.

- Compartment pressures should be measured with a dedicated compartment pressure monitor or an arterial pressure monitoring line
- Fasciotomy must be open, be four-compartment and must be full-length

CHAPTER 3

BURNS, COLD AND SOFT TISSUE INJURIES

BURNS

Background

Approximately 1% of the population suffers a major thermal injury each year, with ~10% requiring hospitalization and ~10% of those having life-threatening injuries.

- Concomitant non-thermal injuries occur in ~5% of burn patients
- The extremes of age (young and old) are at increased risk of burn injuries
- Flame burns are most common in adults whilst scald injuries are most common in children

> Child abuse must be *suspected* for unusual burns in children, when the history does not match the presentation, when the history continually changes, or when there is a delayed presentation

Burn centre transfer criteria

> Appropriate transfer maximizes survival and optimizes outcome; it should be guided by advice from the receiving burn centre

Transfer criteria to a dedicated burn centre
a. Partial-thickness burns >10% total body surface area (TBSA)
b. Full-thickness burns >5% TBSA
c. Any burn requiring fluid resuscitation
d. Burns involving the face, hands, feet, genitalia, perineum or major joints
e. Circumferential burns of the extremities or torso
f. Proven or suspected inhalation injuries
g. Electrical injuries (including lightning)
h. Chemical injuries
i. Burns in patients with significant pre-existing medical conditions or special social, emotional or long-term rehabilitation needs which could complicate management
j. Burns in patients with associated non-thermal trauma

This represents a consolidation of American Burn Association (ABA), European Burn Association (EBA) and Australian & New Zealand Burn Association (ANZBA) criteria. Local Burn Centre policies may differ and local policies should be followed

Complete documentation should follow the patient, with particular emphasis on vital signs, the amount of intravenous (i.v.) fluid administered, and hourly urine output.

Initial management of the burn patient
Management begins with a full history of the mechanism of injury, including

- Type of burn (e.g. flame, scald, chemical, etc.)
- Duration of exposure
- Time of injury (for calculating start time of fluid resuscitation)
- Possibility of inhalation injury (see below) and presence of toxic materials (e.g. plastics, cyanide, petroleum products)
- Possibility of concomitant non-thermal injuries, which must be ruled out, *and* the patient's health before injury, as these greatly influence outcome

Patients with severe burns may appear deceptively stable on arrival, but can quickly become critically ill

Signs and symptoms of inhalation injury
- History of being in a closed space fire
- Carbon deposits in the nasopharynx or oropharynx
- Expectorated carbonaceous sputum
- Wheezing or change in phonation
- PaO_2:FiO_2 <300
- Carbon monoxide levels estimated >10% at the scene

 Supplemental oxygen should be provided to all patients

Estimating burn severity

The percentage of the total body surface area (%TBSA) of any burn is best estimated by the rule of nines in adults or age-appropriate diagrams in children (Fig. 3.1).

Terminology for burn depth using 'degree' has been replaced by the description of 'thickness'.

Burn depth
- Superficial ('first-degree')
  — confined to epidermis with negligible tissue damage
  — mild erythema, pain resolving in 48–72 h
  — epidermis may peel in small scales without scarring

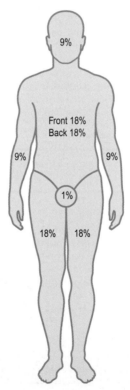

Figure 3.1 Brund and Wallace chart rule of 9s (Adult)

- Partial-thickness ('second-degree')
  — involves entire epidermis with variable layers of dermis
    a. Superficial
  — painful, pink and blistered
    b. Deep
  — red or mottled with minimal/no capillary refill, often dry, ± blisters
  — pinprick perceived as pressure rather than pain

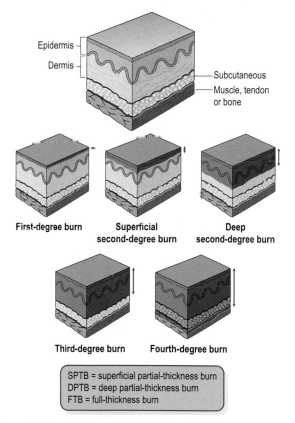

Figure 3.2 Schematic of skin burn depth

- Full-thickness ('third-degree')
  — entire epidermis and dermis destroyed
  — relatively painless
  — leathery, waxy, or charred, sometimes with visible thrombosed vessels

Only partial- and full-thickness injuries contribute to the TBSA estimation that will ultimately guide resuscitation

Burn resuscitation
- Provide early pain control with frequent small doses of i.v. opiates
- Elevate the ambient room temperature to avoid heat loss
- Burns require tetanus prophylaxis

Although urgent endotracheal intubation is sometimes necessary, there is usually time to perform a semi-elective intubation if there are signs and symptoms of inhalation injury

- i.v. access is ideally obtained with two large-bore (14–16-gauge in adults) peripheral catheters, preferably placed through unburnt tissue
- In severe burns (>25% TBSA), central venous access may be required and should be obtained early before massive swelling and oedema occur
- Typically, only burns >15–20% TBSA require formal i.v. fluid resuscitation in adults and >10–15% TBSA in children

- Lactated Ringers (LR, or Hartmann's solution) is the resuscitation fluid of choice
- *Do not use normal saline!!!*
- Some burn units recommend the use of hypertonic saline or early colloid administration to limit volumes of crystalloid resusucitation (be aware of local policies)

- Too much fluid can be as damaging and dangerous as too little
- Over resuscitation can result in compartment syndromes and pulmonary oedema

Adult resuscitation
Parkland/Baxter formula = 4 ml LR/kg body weight/% TBSA burn over 24 h

Give one-half of the calculated requirement in the first 8 h from the time of injury (not when the patient presents). The other half is given over subsequent 16 h
Paediatric resuscitation (infants and toddlers <30 kg)
Modified Parkland/Baxter formula = 3 ml LR/kg body weight/% TBSA burn over 24 h plus weight-based dextrose maintenance fluid requirements
NB Only partial- and full-thickness injuries contribute to the TBSA estimation

Formulae are only guides to initial resuscitation volumes, and fluid rates should be adjusted according to the patient's response.

- Urine output is used to guide adequacy of fluid resuscitation
- Aim for ~30 ml/h in an adult or 1 ml/kg/h in a child, and titrate the fluid resuscitation accordingly

A subset of patients (those with inhalation injury, high voltage electrical, delayed resuscitation or massive deep burns) may require additional fluid over that estimated by the Parkland/Baxter formula.

- Haemoconcentration (i.e. haematocrit >55%) may be an early clue to increased fluid requirements
- Adequacy of fluid resuscitation is still assessed by urine output
- Invasive central monitoring is really only useful in a small subset of patients
  — typically those with a history of severe cardiopulmonary disease
- In the second 24 h post-burn, a patient's maintenance fluid requirements are ~1.5 times normal
  — this volume should be given as crystalloid, with the composition of the fluid determined by serum electrolyte levels
  — colloid supplementation typically occurs ≥24 h post-burn

Initial wound management

- Systemic prophylactic antibiotics are *never* indicated in burn injury!

- In the emergency department, before transfer to a burn centre
  — wash gently with gauze soaked in saline
  — remove any obviously loose skin
  — apply topical agents (see below) only if anticipated delay in transfer
  — irrigate debris from the eyes, as needed
  — cover wounds with dry, non-adhesive dressings (e.g. gauze, cellophane wrap, etc.) or cover the patient with a 'burn sheet'

Topical antimicrobial agents

Silver sulfadiazine 1% cream
- Most common topical agent used on burn wounds
- Usually applied daily or twice daily in a thin layer, followed by wrapping loosely with sterile non-adhesive dressing
- Broad-spectrum, bacteriostatic, antifungal activity
- Painless and usually soothing
- Transient neutropenia (?sulfa-effect) can occur; this is of no clinical consequence
- Caution must be taken in pregnancy and very small infants (<2 months)

Mafenide acetate cream or 5% solution
- Penetrates eschar, somewhat painful (cream much more so than solution)
- Clinically inconsequential, mild metabolic acidosis (carbonic anhydrase inhibitor)
- Broad-spectrum, bacteriostatic, no antifungal activity

Bacitracin ointment
- Ointment (not cream) usually applied to small superficial burns and surfaces difficult to cover with gauze (e.g. face)
- May require several applications per day
- Primarily bacteriostatic against Gram-positive organisms
- Neosporin, polysporin or gentamicin ointments can be substituted for broader bacterial coverage

Acticoat
- Silver-impregnated membrane
- Left in place on the wound for 2–7 days, depending on the formulation

Silver nitrate 0.5% solution
- Broad-spectrum, bacteriostatic, antifungal activity
- Costly, messy and electrolyte abnormalities (e.g. hyponatraemia)

Escharotomy

- Circumferential full-thickness or deep partial-thickness burns of the trunk or extremities can cause compartment syndromes

Indications for escharotomy
- Increased ventilatory pressures in circumferential torso burns
- Decreased distal perfusion or diminished/absent pulses in a circumferential extremity burn

- Contact should be made with the receiving burn centre regarding the need and timing of escharotomies
- Unless transport to definitive centre is to be delayed up to 12 h, escharotomies should be done at the burn centre

Technique
- In theory, this technique is bloodless and painless (usually not the case)
  — provide adequate and appropriate analgesia with sedation
  — perform with electrocautery (preferably), or scalpel with topical haemostatic agents, e.g. Avitene)
- Divide only the eschar, not the subcutaneous tissues or fascia
- Appropriate sites for escharotomy extend along the medial and lateral midaxial lines of the extremities and the midaxillary lines and bilateral subcostal lines of the torso; digital escharotomies are unnecessary
- Inadequate haemostasis with multiple escharotomies can result in clinically significant blood loss

Chemical burns

Most chemical burns are from acids or alkalis, with alkalis generally producing more severe burns secondary to liquefactive (alkali) vs. coagulative (acid) necrosis.

Concentration of the agent and duration of contact influence severity of injury

Tissue damage is frequently underestimated and, unlike thermal burns, continues until the causative agent is removed.

All chemical burns should be copiously irrigated with tepid tap water for at least 15 min (avoid hypothermia); alkali injuries may require up to 1 h of irrigation.

Litmus paper can be useful to establish an endpoint (neutral skin pH).

No specific antidote is available for most chemical burns and neutralizers are contraindicated.

For hydrofluoric acid burns, copiously irrigate and apply calcium gluconate gel.

If indicated, administer intra-venous calcium gluconate.

Electrical injury

- Classified as either high voltage (>1000 V) or low voltage (<1000 V)
- In general, alternating current (AC) is more dangerous than direct current (DC)
- Small skin wounds can hide substantial underlying muscle and bony destruction, particularly with high voltage injuries
- ECG monitoring is only useful in those who have abnormal ECGs on presentation or who have had a cardiac arrest at the scene
- Concomitant muscle damage and potential myoglobinuria may necessitate a higher rate of resuscitation fluid (≥4 ml/kg/% TBSA) to generate higher hourly urine outputs to avoid acute renal failure

FURTHER READING

Holmes J H 4th and Heimbach D M 2005 Burns. In: Brunicardi C F, Andersen D K, Billiar T R et al (eds) Schwartz's principles of surgery, 8th edn. McGraw–Hill, New York

Sheridan R L 2002 Burns. Critical Care Medicine 30(suppl):S500-S514

COLD INJURIES: HYPOTHERMIA AND FROSTBITE

Definition

A core temperature below 35°C (95.0°F)

- Mild: 35–32°C
- Moderate: 32–30°C
- Severe: <30°C

PRIMARY HYPOTHERMIA (TABLE 3.1)

- Caused by a *physiologically normal* patient being exposed to a *cold environment* for a prolonged time

TABLE 3.1 Physiological and metabolic response to cold

	32–35°C (89–95°F)	30–32°C (86–89°F)	<30°C (86°F)
Systemic	↑Oxygen consumption, metabolic acidosis, shivering	↓Oxygen consumption, shivering ceases	
Neurological	EEG abnormal, lethargy, flat affect	Decreased mentation, motor function, reasoning, hyperreflexia	EEG flat, hyporeflexia, hallucinations, stupor, coma
Cardiovascular	Tachycardia, vasoconstriction	Bradycardia, ↓mean arterial pressure, ↓cardiac contractility, ↓CO, EKG-J wave	Increased risk of ventricular fibrillation
Respiratory	↓Respiratory rate, hypoventilation, ↑CO₂, hypoxia, respiratory acidosis	Mucociliary dysfunction	
Coagulation	↓Enzymatic activity 40%, ↓platelet count and function		

- Recognized initially in the military when soldiers were exposed to cold temperatures for extended periods
- Now seen in the civilian population among the homeless, and adventurers into the wilderness

Moderators of the extent of cold injury
- Ambient temperature
- Length of exposure
- Wind chill
- Wet clothing
- Alcohol consumption (vasodilatation and judgement impairment)
- Smoking (vasoconstriction of digits)

Who is most at risk? Men 30–49 years of age (likely the adventuring population)

Some patients may present with hypothermia owing to homes without heating instead of homelessness

Resuscitation/immediate management
- *<C>* Address compelling source of haemorrhage
- *A*irway and *B*reathing are similar to any other resuscitation
  — theoretical risk of precipitating ventricular fibrillation with endotracheal intubation
- *C*irculation, on the other hand, is somewhat modified (Fig. 3.3)
  — if any organized cardiac rhythm exists, *no CPR*, even without a pulse

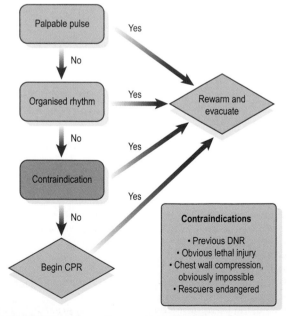

Figure 3.3 Pathway for cardiac resuscitation in hypothermic patient

— CPR is ineffective at cold temperatures because of chest wall
and cardiac muscle rigidity
— in fact, it can be detrimental (i.e. tissue injury, or initiation of
ventricular fibrillation)
— additionally, faint pulses can be difficult to palpate in a cold,
stiff patient

> Because of the substantially decreased metabolic rate
> during hypothermia, some patients may be successfully
> resuscitated even after prolonged cardiac arrest!

Investigation and diagnosis

- History and temperature essentially diagnose this injury
- Many patients will present with cool, pale skin (secondary to
vasoconstriction)
- The secondary survey is extremely important to identify other
associated injuries

> *Beware*: **some clinical thermometers do not read below**
> **35°C (95°F)**

Definitive management

- Therapeutic goals for the hypothermic patient
  - prevent further heat loss
  - prevent ventricular fibrillation
  - rewarm the patient, core prior to shell (or inside before
  outside)
- *Prevention of further heat loss* is achieved by moving the
patient to a neutral ambient temperature, removing wet clothing
and surrounding the patient with warm blankets, especially the
head
- *Prevention of ventricular fibrillation* is best achieved by
electrolyte and volume correction, maintenance of normal CO_2
and avoiding unnecessary CPR
- In the event of ventricular fibrillation, cardiac drugs and
defibrillation should not be used until core temperature is greater
than 28°C
- *Rewarming*
  - core rewarming is the most effective management for
  hypothermia

Rewarming techniques (Table 3.2)
- Passive, using the patient's own metabolic heat to raise core temperature while insulating the dry patient at a room temperature of 25–33°C (77–91°F)
  — acceptable only for mildly hypothermic patients (>33°C or 91°F) and only if not otherwise compromised by the hypothermia
- Active, administering internal or external heat to warm the patient
  — external devices such as warming blankets, lamps or warm water immersion are acceptable for the moderately hypothermic patient (30–32°C or 89–95°F), but are generally ineffective, and potentially detrimental, to those who are severely hypothermic
  — warm fluids, warm humidified ventilation gases, warm fluid lavage of body cavities (chest, abdomen)

> If available, cardiopulmonary bypass should be used in patients with severe hypothermia (<30°C or 89°F), or in those who have clinical compromise such as cardiac arrest, frostbite or rhabdomyolysis. If bypass is not available, alternative active strategies as outlined above should be continued

 No patient is dead until they are warm and dead

SECONDARY HYPOTHERMIA

Definition
Systemic hypothermia which develops in a *physiologically compromised* patient in a *normothermic* environment.

- This much more common type of hypothermia is most often demonstrated in the exsanguinating trauma patient and is often identified by dysfunction of the coagulation system during operation. Other diseases such as alcoholism, endocrine dysfunction and cardiovascular disease can put patients at risk of hypothermia in relatively warm environments
- Therapy is rewarming, although the lowest temperature nadir is rarely as extreme as with primary hypothermia. Other systemic

TABLE 3.2 Systemic response to rewarming techniques in hypothermia

	Passive	Intravenous fluids	Airway	Peritoneal lavage	Cardiopulmonary bypass
Substrate temperature (°C)	25–33	40	40–45	40–45	
Rate of rewarming (°C/h)	0.5–2	0.14 per litre	1–2	2–4	1–2°C q 3–5 min

therapies such as replacement of blood products lost during haemorrhage, as well as correction of volume depletion (all fluids should be warmed), are crucial in this type of hypothermia

 Hypothermia can occur in a room that feels warm!

FROSTBITE

Definition
Freezing injury to the periphery with ice crystal formation in the interstitium resulting in cellular desiccation: usually hands, feet, ears and nose.

> Why are humans susceptible to frostbite while many animals who live, unprotected in the cold, don't get frostbite? The autoregulation of peripheral vascular beds which contributes to core warming (and peripheral hypoperfusion) is unique to humans

Clinical presentation
- Systemic injury or hypothermia are often present
- Affected areas are initially blanched and waxy-appearing, with blisters with clear or milky fluid. More severely injured tissues have haemorrhagic fluid in the blisters, or are firm and covered with eschar. Erythema and oedema may be present if tissue thawing has already ensued. The extent of tissue injury is very difficult to discern for weeks

Therapy (Table 3.3)
- Treat systemic hypothermia and injuries first
- Rewarm in warm water at a temperature of 39–42°C (102–108°F) until flushing returns (usually approximately 30 min)
- Fasciotomy is undertaken if compartment syndrome is suspected
- Clear blisters should be debrided to reduce wound contact with prostaglandins and thromboxanes in blister fluid which cause vasoconstriction and platelet aggregation
- Haemorrhagic blisters are not debrided

TABLE 3.3 Management of frostbite wounds			
Field	*Acute*	*Subacute*	*Long term*
Immediate	Initial contact with hospital	1st 3–4 weeks	1–3 months
Protective dressing, but do not warm	Rewarm in water bath	Protective dressings and direct wound care	Debridement or amputation based on demarcation

- Systemic ibuprofen and topical aloe vera may decrease the platelet aggregation and vasoconstriction caused by prostaglandins and thromboxanes
- Cleanse daily in whirlpool
- Elevate extremity
- Use protective tent to avoid additional injury
- Keep extremity dry to avoid maceration
- Begin mobilization when oedema has resolved and blisters have desiccated
- No smoking
- Tetanus immunization
- Use antibiotics only for identified infectious complications; prophylactic antibiotics are not indicated

It is important to protect affected areas from repeated exposures because previously frostbitten tissues are more cold-sensitive; they are thus at higher risk of frostbite at otherwise non-threatening temperatures

TRENCHFOOT/CHILBLAINS

Definition
Chronic exposure to cold (not freezing) and damp conditions resulting in loss of function of tissue due to ischaemia from vasoconstriction and neurological injury due to myelin sheath degradation.

Investigation and diagnosis
Cold, painful feet with waxy or, after hyperaemia, erythematous with blister formation and pruritis.

Definitive management

Warming, gently washing, drying, elevation.

FURTHER READING

Long W B, Edlich R F, Winters K L et al 2005 Cold Injuries. Journal of
Long-term Effect of Medical Implants 15(1):67–78

Petrone P, Kuncir E J, Asensio J A 2003 Surgical management and strategies
in the treatment of hypothermia and cold injury. Emergency Medical
Clinics of North America 21:1165–1178

Reed II R L, Gentilello L M 2004 Temperature-associated injuries and
syndromes. In: Moore E E, Feliciano D V, Mattox K L (eds) Trauma, 5th
edn. McGraw–Hill, New York, p 1099–1107

SOFT TISSUE INJURIES

Background

Soft tissue injuries are common in major trauma. In general, most
soft tissue injuries are dealt with in the secondary and tertiary
surveys. It is important that these injuries are detected and
managed properly. This is even more so in the multiple trauma
setting, as there is a high rate of missed injuries in this group; this
is higher still in those with blunt trauma. This will contribute not
only to the morbidity but also mortality of patients. The adoption
of a tertiary survey as a matter of routine within 24 h and before
discharge will decrease the level of these missed injuries (see section
on Tertiary Survey).

It is rare for soft tissue injuries to be directly life- or
limb-threatening, but in these cases it is important to pre-empt this
and institute emergency management to minimize mortality and
morbidity rates.

POTENTIALLY LIFE-THREATENING SOFT TISSUE INJURIES

Crush syndrome

It is vital to recognize and pre-empt this condition, which is
characterized by the clinical picture of:

- Hypovolaemia
- Muscle breakdown
- High potassium
- Renal failure

Failure to recognize that crush injury is present can cause a rapid deterioration in clinical status, leading to death. It may occur in patients who remain trapped. These patients characteristically appear to remain stable while still crushed, only to rapidly deteriorate once the pressure is released.

- Pre-emptive treatment with fluid boluses and an aggressive management strategy to monitor for, and counteract the effects of, hyperkalaemia are vital
- The crushed tissues sequestrate fluid, causing fluid depletion which exacerbates the direct toxic effect of released myoglobins on the kidneys

Management <C>
- Adherence to <C> ABCDE principles
- Aggressive fluid resuscitation is needed
- Check for urine myoglobins
- Check serum potassium
  — dextrose/insulin and i.v. calcium gluconate
- Monitor the ECG for changes associated with high potassium
  — peaked waves
  — widened QRS, etc.
- Alkalinization of urine can be considered

Gas gangrene
Gas gangrene is a potentially life-threatening condition. It is caused by an exotoxin-producing *Clostridium* (the commonest cause in 90% is *Cl. perfringens*); these bacteria are routinely present in the soil and gastrointestinal tract. Although rare, it carries a mortality rate approaching 25%.

> **Risk factors**
> Immunocompromise, diabetes, peripheral vascular disease and drug abuse

The history is characteristically of an injury which, within 72 h, is associated with toxaemia and pain that seems to be in excess of physical findings.

- Clinical findings include
  — the presence of bullae
  — crepitus
  — brawny oedema
  — foul sweet-smelling discharge

Management <C>

- Adherence to ABCDEs
- High flow oxygen is needed
- Toxaemic patients will be hypovolaemic and will need aggressive fluid resuscitation
- The early administration of antibiotics (see below), together with involvement of the critical care and surgical team, is vital to decrease mortality rates
- Aggressive surgical debridement is the mainstay of treatment
- Antibiotics
  — penicillin plus an aminoglycoside
  — clindamycin in the penicillin-allergic patient

Tetanus

This is caused by *Clostridium tetani*, a Gram-positive anaerobic rod bacterium found in soil, and human and animal faeces. It is heat-sensitive and cannot survive in oxygen, hence its predilection for devitalized tissues. It produces its effects through tetanolysin and tetanospasmin, which is a potent neurotoxin.

Tetanus prophylaxis

New guidelines were issued in 2002 to cover the prophylaxis of tetanus since Tettox is now combined with diphtheria. The following summary will guide management (Table 3.4). Further information is available in the Green Book (Immunizations against Infectious Diseases) or on the Department of Health website www.dh.gov.uk

POTENTIALLY LIMB-THREATENING INJURIES

Degloving injuries

These injuries cause traction injuries to the nerves and to the blood supply.

Amputations

Amputations occur as a result of industrial and agricultural accidents but can also occur in other forms of trauma. Traumatic amputations can be partial or complete, when there remains a bridge of tissue. Often the mangled crush type of amputation bleeds less (owing to the local tissue damage, which induces a marked vasospasm).

Viability of reimplantation needs to be assessed by a specialist in this field. In principle, cleancut amputations and those that

TABLE 3.4 Requirement for tetanus prophylaxis following injury

Current immunization status	Vaccine	Immunoglobulin	Vaccine
Full (five injections)	No	No	Only if high risk
Up to date but not yet achieved five injections	No (unless nearly due and more convenient)	No (unless nearly due and more convenient)	Only if high risk
Primary immunizations not completed or not up to date	Yes (and ensure completed course arranged)	Yes (and ensure course completed)	Yes
Not immunized Unknown status	Yes (and arrange full course if needed)	Yes (and include full course if indicated)	Yes

are more distal do better. It is important that parts are kept in a condition to offer the best chance of using them; occasionally they may even be used as a potential for grafts.

NON-LIFE-THREATENING SOFT TISSUE INJURY

Most trauma victims will sustain a range of 'minor' soft tissue injuries in addition to their major injuries; these include abrasions, contusions and lacerations. Many of these will only come to light following the initial resuscitation, during the secondary and tertiary surveys, and significant bruising may continue to develop for some time after the initial injury. Occasionally these injuries can be significant.

All soft tissue injuries need to be assessed, accurately recorded and managed appropriately.

CHAPTER 4

SPECIAL PHYSIOLOGY

INJURED ELDERLY

Background
With the improvements in healthcare, people are living active lives well into their seventh and eighth decades.

This rapid population growth, combined with the fact that elderly trauma patients utilize *one-third* of all trauma-related expenses, poses a substantial challenge to trauma care providers.

Essentials

> **Physiological age is more important than chronological age**

- Age: the mortality rate increases by 5% each year for patients >65 years old
- Pre-existing conditions/comorbidities
- 33% of patients 65 years and older have at least one chronic pre-existing condition
- The presence of a pre-existing condition increases mortality rates between two and eight times that of an uninjured cohort for up to 5 years after injury
- Comorbidities have the greatest detrimental effect in less severely injured patients
  — when injury severity score (ISS)>25, outcome is a function of injury severity
- Decreased physiological reserve equates to an inability to respond to the stress of injury and results in the patient being more likely to develop complications
- Complications increase mortality rates
  — one complication leads to an 8.6% increase, and two complications to more than a 30% increase in mortality rate

Physiological effects of ageing
- Renal
  — reduction of renal mass 30–40%
  — inability to concentrate urine and conserve water leads to chronic dehydration
- Thermoregulation
  — less efficient heat conservation/production owing to lower lean tissue mass
  — increased oxygen consumption and cardiac demands because of shivering

- Respiratory
  — loss of muscular strength and endurance
  — decreased chest wall compliance
  — impaired secretion clearance because of cilia dysmotility
- Cardiovascular
  — decreased response to endogenous catecholamines leads to lower cardiac output, ejection fraction and maximal heart rate
  — coronary atherosclerosis decreases diastolic filling during tachycardia and hypotension
- CNS
  — cerebral atrophy results in an increase in the subdural space
  — cognitive changes in memory and judgement
  — depressed sensory acquisition (visual, auditory, proprioception)
- Musculoskeletal
  — bone density loss results in skeletal fragility
  — decreased lean muscle mass and serum creatinine production

> A 'normal' admission creatinine is not normal in elderly patients

Mechanism of injury

Blunt trauma
Blunt trauma is overwhelmingly the most common cause of injury in the elderly.

- Falls
  — there were over 3.2 million fall-related injuries in 2003 in the USA
  — each year, over 40% of the elderly in the community and more than 60% of those in nursing homes will sustain a fall
  — are the primary cause of injury and injury-related death in patients >74 years of age
  — are the number 2 cause of injury and injury-related death in patients aged 65–74 years
  — may be due to impaired gait and balance, loss of vision and strength, and comorbidities
- Motor vehicle collisions
  — accounted for over 7000 elderly deaths in 2001 in the USA; this was the second most common cause of death
  — 19 million drivers are >65 years, an increase of 32% since 1991

— are the primary cause of injury and injury-related death in patients aged 65–74 years
— the fatality rate is only second to drivers aged 16–20 years
— usually occur in daylight, weekdays and involve another vehicle
— due to decreased vision and hearing, impaired judgement and delayed reaction times
- Pedestrian
  — 10% of all auto–pedestrian accidents
  — elderly account for 25% of auto–pedestrian fatalities
  — there are higher rates of moderate and severe injuries compared to younger victims
  — mortality rates are in excess of 20%, mostly because of trauma to the brain and thorax
  — greater than 40% of accidents occur at crossings
  — due to impaired gait, reaction times, agility and judgement

Penetrating trauma/assault
- Less common than blunt injury but more lethal
- Elderly only account for 5.7% of victims from intentional trauma
- Mortality rates are five times higher than in the younger population
- Caused by lack of mobility, solitary lifestyle and inability to defend oneself

Burns
- Elderly burn victims account for 20% of burn unit admissions
- Burns account for 8% of trauma-related elderly fatalities
- Injury patterns are usually larger and deeper burns owing to chronic epidermal atrophy
  — owing to mobility limitations in escape and sensory impairment of fire detection

 A *minor* fall can cause *major* injuries

RESUSCITATION

Early physiological support and identification of life-threatening injuries are primary concerns. Evaluation and treatment of the elderly patient should proceed in an organized and efficient manner following the <C>ABC priorities.

Healthcare providers must be aware of the effects of ageing and comorbidities in the early resuscitation of elderly trauma patients.

<C>Catastrophic haemorrhage
Airway
- Early airway control with intubation should be considered

Breathing
- Poor chest wall compliance and pulmonary reserve leads to physiologically significant 'mild' hypoxia
- Auscultation should determine symmetry of breath sounds and chest wall tenderness should be evaluated
- A 'small' tension pneumothorax can have deleterious effects on cardiac function
- Early pain control for rib fractures will allow for pulmonary optimization, i.e. epidural or intercostal blocks

Circulation
- Early fluid administration augments cardiac function; consider invasive monitoring
- Chronic dehydration and medications limit cardiac response to traumatic injury
- 'Mild' hypotension and tachycardia can lead to myocardial infarction in the diseased heart

Disability
- Rapid detection of neurological impairment should be performed
- Cerebral atrophy allows for a longer 'lucent' period with intracranial bleeding
- Spinal stenosis and osteophyte formation results in spinal cord injury with minor falls

Exposure
- Complete exposure is vital
- Evaluation of previous surgical scars may provide significant medical history which may be otherwise unobtainable, i.e. median sternotomy, lumbar surgery, peripheral vascular disease

- Confusion is caused by impaired cerebral oxygenation until proven otherwise, not dementia
- Beta-blockers will maintain a 'normal' heart rate during shock
- A neurological deficit is due to an (extra) epidural or subdural haematoma until proven otherwise, not a previous stroke
- Early fluid resuscitation augments oxygen delivery during the stress response and will not cause acute congestive heart failure

Outcomes

- Elderly trauma patients have three to four times higher mortality and morbidity rates than their younger counterparts
- Age alone conveys a 5% increase in mortality for each year beyond 65
- In severe injury, outcome is more dependent on injury severity than comorbidities
- At low to moderate injury severity, pre-existing comorbidities have significant impact on the outcome
    — hepatic, renal and cardiac disease before injury are the most significant independent predictors of mortality, increasing the risk of death by between two and eight times
- An elderly patient in a ground level fall sustains as much traumatic injury as a fall from height in a younger patient
    — this 'minor' mechanism of trauma warrants a complete trauma evaluation and possible hospital admission
- Early aggressive intervention with fluid resuscitation and invasive monitoring in an intensive care unit (ICU) setting is justified in patients with multiple comorbidities, severe injury or hypotension
- With early goal-directed resuscitation, mortality rates have been reduced from 93% to 47%

The residual effects of traumatic injury in the elderly population last long after hospital discharge. Equal numbers of patients are discharged from an inpatient hospital setting to home, short-term rehabilitation and skilled nursing facilities (SNF).

- A return to independent living is achieved in 63% of elderly trauma victims
- Patients over 80 years of age more often require rehabilitation or SNF at discharge

- This population most often has deficits in mobility and activities of daily living; however, their ability for social interaction and expression remains intact
- Over time, 50% of patients discharged to a SNF will return home with assistance

Special considerations
- Blunt splenic injury
  — conservative non-operative management is successful in 80% of patients
  — elderly patients fail conservative management more frequently than younger patients
  — failed conservative management results in increased mortality and morbidity rates in the elderly population
  — higher failure rates are seen with contrast extravasation on CT scan, high grade of splenic injury, combined hepatic and splenic injuries, and multiple transfusions
  — based on limited physiological reserve, early splenectomy may be indicated
- Central cord syndrome
  — spinal stenosis increases the risk of central cord syndrome
  — often associated with cervical hyperextension from forward ground level falls
  — neurological deficits are seen in the upper extremities, with lower extremity sparing
  — occurs without cervical spine fracture. CT or MRI is essential for diagnosis
  — prognosis for full functional recovery is poor, with mortality rates in excess of 50%
- Anticoagulation
  — anticoagulation medication is used by >15% of the elderly population
  — patients with an elevated prothrombin time and intracranial bleed have worse outcomes
  — rapid utilization of head CT with even minor head trauma is indicated
  — if pathology is present, reversal with fresh frozen plasma and admission to the ICU are indicated
  — appropriate reversal of antiplatelet medications in the setting of traumatic brain injury is not yet supported by the literature

FURTHER READING

Grossman M D, Miller D, Scaff D W et al 2002 When is an elder old? Effect of preexisting conditions on mortality in geriatric trauma. Journal of Trauma 52:242–246

Kauder D R 1998 Geriatric trauma. In: Peitzman A B, Rhodes M, Schwab C W et al (eds) The Trauma Manual. Lippincott–Raven, Philadelphia, p 469–477

McGwin G, MacLennan P A, Fife J B et al 2004 Preexisting conditions and mortality in older trauma patients. Journal of Trauma 56:1291–1296

Schwab C W, Shapiro M B, Kauder D R 2000 Geriatric trauma: patterns, care, and outcomes. In: Mattox K L, Feliciano D V, Moore E E (eds) Trauma, 4th edn. McGraw–Hill, New York, p 1041–1059

YOUNG PATIENTS—PAEDIATRIC INJURY

Background

Trauma is the leading cause of morbidity, mortality and years of potential life lost for children in the industrialized world. There are anatomical, physiological and mechanistic differences which must be considered when caring for the paediatric trauma patient. Understanding these differences and developing an appropriate knowledge base is essential for all trauma care providers, as many adult centres report that up to 25% of their population is paediatric.

Essentials

- Paediatric trauma resuscitation follows the same <C>ABC guidelines and principles as are applied to the adult trauma victim
- Anatomical differences unique to the child will impact on the trauma management
- The physiological response to injury differs in children and will impact on management of the injuries
- The specific injuries sustained by children may differ from those in adults despite similar injury mechanisms

Airway

Anatomical differences

- Large occiput (when supine causes flexion of the neck and occlusion of the airway)
- High larynx, short trachea, posterior epiglottis
- Newborns are obligate nasal breathers (avoid occluding nares with tubes and clear secretions or blood as necessary)

- Large tongue may occlude airway
- Airway narrowing at cricoid cartilage (use uncuffed endotracheal tube)

Initial airway management
- Establish patient airway (sniffing position, chin lift, jaw thrust, clear oropharynx of debris)
- Provide supplemental oxygen in all cases
- Insert oral airway (if indicated)
- Intubate trachea (if indicated; orotracheal route preferred)

Endotracheal intubation
- Utilize rapid sequence intubation techniques
- Use uncuffed endotracheal tube whenever possible in younger children (<8 years)
- Estimate appropriate tube size by: diameter of external nares, diameter of smallest finger, or using the formula: $(age/4) + 4$
- *Always* confirm appropriate position of tube by auscultation of both lung fields, observation of chest wall movement and capnography. Record position by chest radiograph and capnography

Breathing
- The most common cause of cardiac arrest in paediatric trauma patients is hypoventilation
- Look for signs of respiratory insufficiency: muscular retractions, nasal flaring, grunting, extreme anxiety
- For persistent hypoventilation assess for: pneumothorax, mainstem intubation, oesophageal intubation, tracheobronchial injury, pulmonary contusion

Circulation
- Recognition of shock in the child may be difficult (or delayed) because of a robust compensatory physiology
- Recognize abnormal vital signs (Table 4.1)
- Recognize features of shock (Table 4.2); tachycardia is the first sign, hypotension a late sign
- Begin volume resuscitation early (10–20 ml/kg normal saline boluses)
- Move to blood product replacement if no response to crystalloid therapy

Resuscitation is dynamic—reassess response to therapy frequently

TABLE 4.1 Normal vital signs by age

Age (years)	Heart rate (bpm)	Systolic blood pressure (mmHg)	Respiratory rate (breaths/min)
0–1	<180	>60	<60
1–3	<160	>70	<40
3–6	<140	>75	<35
6–12	<120	>90	<30
>12	<100	>90–100	<20

TABLE 4.2 Clinical features of shock in the paediatric patient

	Cardiac	Mental status	Skin (perfusion)	Renal
<25% blood volume	Thready pulse, including heart rate	Lethargic and confused	Cool and clammy	Decreased urine output, including specific gravity
25–50% blood volume	Pronounced increase in heart rate	Diminished level of consciousness, dulled response to pain	Cyanosis and delayed capillary refill	Minimal urine output
>50% blood volume of blood lost	Pronounced increase in heart rate, hypotension	Comatose	Pale and cold	No urine output

Disability

- Rapid assessment of level of consciousness, pupil size and reactivity is required
- Note extremity movement, tone and reflexes
- Determine Glasgow Coma Score (GCS; Table 4.3)

Exposure

- Completely undress and evaluate entire body
- Keep warm!
- Check under collars and splints

TABLE 4.3 GCS scores for infant and non-infant patients

	Adult			Infant	
Activity	Response	Score	Activity	Response	Score
Eye opening	Spontaneous	4	Eye opening	Spontaneous	4
	To verbal	3		To verbal	3
	To pain	2		To pain	2
	None	1		None	1
Verbal	Oriented	5	Verbal	Coos, babbles	5
	Confused	4		Irritable crying	4
	Inappropriate	3		Cries to pain	3
	Non-specific	2		Moans to pain	2
	None	1		None	1
Motor	Follows commands	6	Motor	Normal	6
	Localizes pain	5		Withdraws to touch	5
	Withdraws to pain	4		Withdraws to pain	4
	Flexion to pain	3		Flexion to pain	3
	Extension to pain	2		Extension to pain	2
	None	1		None	1

- Logroll, examine back
- Rectal examination
- Re-cover as soon as possible to prevent hypothermia

Special considerations

Venous access
- Often a challenging aspect of resuscitation
- Establish a defined time limit for peripheral access attempts
- If in shock, move to intraosseus or central access early
- Site of central access (e.g. femoral, subclavian) determined by practitioner experience
- Intraosseus access relatively easy and reliable for younger children (<6 years)
  — suitable for volume, medications and blood products
  — intraosseus access is temporary: establish additional access as resuscitation progresses
  — use the anteromedial surface, 1–3 cm below the tibial tuberosity; direct away from the growth plate and do not place below a fracture site

HEAD INJURY

- Most common cause of fatal injury in the paediatric age group
- Fontanelles and sutures may protect from raised intracranial pressure (ICP) until late in course
- Patients may lose a significant amount of blood into the epidural or subgaleal spaces
- Consider ICP monitoring for GCS<8
- Prevent secondary brain injury (hypoxia, oedema)

THORACIC INJURY

- This is the second most common site of fatal injury in injured children
- Rib fractures are less common owing to increased compliance
    — more energy is transmitted to underlying structures, thus pulmonary contusion is relatively more common
- Greater mediastinal mobility may result in tension physiology with pneumothorax
- Overall, the need for operative intervention for thoracic injury is uncommon

ABDOMINAL INJURY

- This is the third most common site of fatal injury in children and the most common site of occult fatal injury
- Remember to decompress the stomach and bladder
- Larger organs, lax musculature and compliant ribs lead to increased risk to abdominal organs
- The abdomen extends to nipple level with deep exhalation
- CT scan is the current gold standard for evaluation of the paediatric abdomen
- Solid organ injuries (kidney, liver, spleen) are commonly managed non-operatively
    — this approach is a trade-off of risk of early, operative complications (haemorrhage, coagulopathy and death) for possible later complications (infection or perforation)
    — successful in most series for >90% of cases, including high grade injuries
    — safe (with appropriate monitoring) for multiple solid organ injuries, and with associated head injury
    — low threshold to reimage; recognize failure

SPINAL CORD INJURY

- Comparatively less common in children
- Proportionately larger head and lax ligaments may result in increased force applied to the neck
- Consider spinal cord injury without radiological abnormality (SCIWORA)
- Pseudosubluxation of C2 on C3 is seen in 40% of normal children up to age 7 years, and 20% up to age 16 years
- The use of high-dose steroids for spinal cord injuries in children remains controversial and should be dictated by local practice

MUSCULOSKELETAL INJURY

- Variety of fractures unique to the paediatric population
- Injuries to the growth plate may result in long-term disability
- Children may sequester a proportionately greater amount of blood with fractures (particularly the femur) compared to adults
- Vascular injuries are associated with specific fracture types (e.g. supracondylar humeral fracture)
- Radiographs are often difficult to interpret owing to normal growth plates; comparison to the contralateral side is often helpful

THERMOREGULATION

- The high ratio of body surface area to mass and lower fat content put children (particularly infants) at risk for hypothermia
- Use warmed i.v. fluids and blood products
- Use heated ventilator circuit, overhead warmer or warming blanket to maintain core temperature

CHILD ABUSE

- Must maintain a high index of suspicion
- Need low threshold to investigate suspicious clinical history or physical findings
- Because of the force associated with child abuse, there is often a high mortality rate
- Child abuse may be the cause of unexplained cardiac arrest

PENETRATING INJURY

- Less common in children (5–15% of the trauma population at most centres)
- Same treatment priorities as adult patients

ENDING THE PAEDIATRIC RESUSCITATION

- There are no well-established guidelines
- Perceived resilience of paediatric patients
- Difficult, emotional decision
- Declare death for:
  - cardiopulmonary resuscitation >20 min (in or out of hospital)
  - asystole
  - pulseless *and* heart rate <40 bpm
- Limited resuscitation for:
  - respiratory arrest
  - pulseless *or* heart rate <40
  - severe hypotension with arrest
  - if intubated in the field
- Emergency department thoracotomy of no value in blunt trauma
- Emergency department thoracotomy of limited value in penetrating trauma

FURTHER READING

Advanced trauma life support for doctors course manual 7th edn 2004 American College of Surgeons, Chicago ATLS
Stafford P W, Blinman T A, Nance M L 2002 Practical points in evaluation and resuscitation of the injured child. Surgical Clinics of North America 82:273–301

OBESITY IN TRAUMA

Background

Obesity is a disease that affects trauma patients in *all* aspects of care. It alters physiology and is associated with many comorbidities. For the same ISS, obese patients have a greater mortality rate than non-obese patients.

Definition

Obesity is somewhat loosely defined. However, it is often characterized by body mass index (BMI). The characterizations are generally as given in Table 4.4.

Remember that BMI = weight (kg)/height (metres)^2

Essentials

- Worldwide at least 1.1 billion people are overweight; 250 million of these are obese
- The incidence of obesity is increasing, as much as doubling in the past 20 years
- Nearly 20% of 18–29 year olds are obese
- Obesity is the leading risk factor for death—ahead of smoking!
- Obesity can increase the 30-year mortality rate by 4–12 times
- Obesity accounts for 12% of the healthcare budget in the USA
- Although obesity is an independent risk factor for death, it is also highly associated with many other disease processes which contribute to death in all populations, including those who are injured

Comorbidities associated with obesity
Hypertension
Dyslipidaemia
Diabetes
Gallbladder disease
Pulmonary dysfunction
Gout
Arthritis
Gastro-oesophageal reflux disease
Coronary artery disease
Left ventricular hypertrophy
Congestive heart failure
Pulmonary hypertension

Injury

- Patients can be difficult to extract from apparently tight areas. Therefore extra workers are often necessary for patient mobilization
- Patients may exceed the weight, or width limitations, of stretchers or ambulances. It is important for emergency medical

TABLE 4.4 Body mass index and obesity	
Body type	*BMI*
Normal	<25
Overweight	25–30
Obese	30–35
Morbidly obese	35–55
Super-morbidly obese	>55

services crews to know those limitations, and to have appropriate alternatives to transportation
- Cervical spine protection must be achieved by methods other than collars (i.e. towels/sandbags taped beside the head)
- Most obese patients will have pulmonary compromise when laying supine
- Difficult intubation is highly correlated with increasing BMI. Patients may arrive with alternative airway protection

Transportation to the emergency department will often be prolonged due to the challenges of extrication from the scene of injury

Resuscitation/immediate management
- In the event of adequate pre-notification, acquire some helpful resources (i.e. a stretcher able to withstand the mass, very experienced intubators, extra lifting/moving resources)
- Once the patient arrives, remember to begin your evaluation using <C>ABC protocols
- If the patient needs to be intubated, have the entire team focus on, and be ready to assist with, this potentially difficult activity
- When rolling the patient for examination, remember that width is often more of a problem than weight. Include multiple caregivers at the bedside

Be prepared to do much of your early care with the obese patient *in the reverse Trendelenberg* position. As soon as it is feasible/safe, move the patient to an *upright* position. Pulmonary compromise from a heavy chest wall and abdomen impinging on the domain of the thoracic cavity will rapidly become your enemy as you attempt to protect this patient from unnecessary intubation

Investigation and diagnosis

- Plain radiographs
  - — it is often difficult to obtain x-rays which sufficiently penetrate the excessive soft tissue for diagnostic decisions
- Ultrasound
  - — much deeper tissues require higher frequency settings and result in poorer definition
- CT/MRI scanning
  - — images are often good, but the power of the table to support large masses and the diameter of the gantry prevent most morbidly obese patients from these imaging techniques
- Angiography
  - — substantial penetration is necessary, much like plain radiography. Additionally, arterial access is more difficult when a large pannus intrudes upon the femoral vasculature

 Key: be creative and flexible with your diagnostic modalities

Definitive management

Ventilator management

- Morbid obesity results in decreased functional residual capacity primarily due to the weight of the chest wall and intrusion from the abdominal cavity
- Normal tidal volumes (5–8 cm^3/kg lean body mass) and elevated positive end expiratory pressure (PEEP = 7–10 cmH$_2$O) are most effectively used in supporting, and safely extubating, these patients

Wound care

- Pressure ulcers are easily acquired in the morbidly obese, and can be fatal
- The challenges of moving these patients, and the high localized pressures, contribute to the incidence of pressure ulcers

Metabolism
- Morbid obesity results in a decreased ability to mobilize or utilize fat, and an increased and, consequently, increased consumption of protein stores after injury
- This is likely to be secondary to elevated glucose and insulin, and decreased catecholamines compared to non-obese injured patients

> Pressure wounds increase by weight over time. Obese patients can develop pressure ulcers extremely rapidly

Safety of caregivers
Each action to be carried out with morbidly obese patients requires planning to arrange an organized effort of movement.

- A simple action such as moving a patient up in bed can result in back strain or losing control of the patient
- The patient should be encouraged to participate in his/her own mobilization if they are able
- Many obese people have been functioning independent of assistance, and were at least somewhat mobile prior to their injury. Their participation will reduce risk to caregivers and improve their convalescence

FURTHER READING

Abir R, Bell R 2004 Assessment and management of the obese patient. Critical Care Medicine 32(4)(suppl):S87–S91

Adams J P, Murphy P G 2000 Obesity in anaesthesia and intensive care. British Journal of Anaesthesia 85(1):91–108

Byrnes M C, McDaniel M D, Moore M B et al 2005 The effect of obesity on outcomes among injured patients. Journal of Trauma 58:232–237

Grant P, Newcombe M 2004 Emergency management of the morbidly obese. Emergency Medicine of Australia 16:309–317

TRAUMA IN PREGNANCY

Background
Trauma is the leading cause of non-obstetric death in women of reproductive age. The Committee on Trauma of the American College of Surgeons estimate that 6% of all pregnancies are complicated by some form of trauma. Trauma is also the

commonest non-obstetric cause of death in pregnancy (up to one in five deaths), with most deaths being from head injury and haemorrhagic shock.

> One in every 300 trauma patients will be pregnant
> There is a 10–20% mortality rate from major trauma in pregnant patients

- It is important to understand the effect of pregnancy on the patient as well as the potential effect of the trauma on the pregnancy
- In maternal shock, 80% of pregnancies will result in fetal death
- Multiple injury and the presence of severe abdominal injury or pelvic fractures are risk factors for fetal death

> Maternal shock causes fetal death in 80% of cases
> Pre-empt and treat shock aggressively

Common causes of trauma in pregnancy
- Blunt trauma (motor vehicle collisions account for two-thirds of all traumas)
- Falls
- Assaults (including domestic violence)
- Burns

 Screen for domestic violence in pregnant assault victims

Clinically important effects of pregnancy on mother (Table 4.5)
- A lot of the changes that occur during pregnancy are designed to protect the mother from blood loss and to oxygenate the fetus effectively
- Uterine blood flow is not autoregulated and is thus sensitive to the sympathetic response—because of this, even before shock is clinically apparent the uterine blood flow may have fallen by 20%
- In the supine pregnant trauma patient the gravid uterus can cause compression of the vena cava, dramatically reducing

TABLE 4.5 Summary of major important changes in pregnancy		
System	*Changes*	*Clinical significance*
Airway	Glottic oedema High risk of regurgitation	Intubation can be difficult Airway is at risk from vomiting/regurgitation
Breathing	Increased respiratory rate Increased minute ventilation Increased tidal volume Raised oxygen consumption Diaphragm pushed up	Pregnancy is a breathless state Provide high flow oxygen to all pregnant patients May need to place chest drains in higher space Desaturation occurs rapidly
Circulation	Relative hypervolaemia (plasma volume increases by 50%) Caval compression when laid flat after 20 weeks Resting heart rate up to 15% higher Pelvic blood flow and venous engorgement means higher pelvic blood flow	Loss of 2 l may have little discernible effect Marked reduction in blood flow unless fetus moved off inferior vena cava Give 2 l of fluid to all pregnant major trauma patients regardless of their apparent haemodynamic status
Disability	AVPU (alert, verbal, pain, unresponsive)	If any response to pain, aim to control airway as soon as possible (including cricoid pressure)
Resuscitation phase	x-rays may damage fetus	See below; x-rays as needed for maternal wellbeing

venous return. These patients should be resuscitated in a left tilt position on the spinal board or by manipulation of the uterus to the left to reduce caval compression

To relieve vena caval compression:
- Left tilt/logroll to left lateral position
- Manual uterine displacement to left

Abdominal investigation in pregnancy
Haemodynamically important liver and splenic injuries are more common in pregnant women suffering major blunt abdominal trauma. In general, diagnostic peritoneal lavage has been largely

TABLE 4.5 *cont'd*

	Secondary survey	
Respiratory	Lower CO_2 Decreased functional residual capacity Increased atelectasis	Watch for hypoventilation Desaturation occurs quickly
Cardiovascular	Cardiac output rises by 40% at 24 weeks Blood pressure	Placental blood flow falls before shock becomes clinically apparent Declines slightly during pregnancy Systolic changes a little Diastolic falls 5–10 mmHg until 36 weeks
Gastrointestinal tract	Reduced motility and gastric emptying Lower oesophageal sphincter tone reduced Uterine pressure on the stomach Uterus displaces organs from their normal position Peritoneum is chronically stretched	Risk of aspiration Early intubation Bowel injury is less common Peritonism may not be clinically as apparent
Haematological	Increase in plasma volume (50%) Increased red cell mass White cell count rises in third trimester Change in coagulability Haematocrit is lower	Physiological anaemia Can be up to 12×10^9 cells/l Risk of deep vein thrombosis Can be as low as 30%
Renal	The bladder becomes extrapelvic after the first trimester	Bladder more susceptible to injury
Anaesthetic drugs	Can suppress beat to beat variability of fetal tracing	Be aware of this when monitoring cardiotocography
CNS	Low CO_2 causes a direct uterine vasoconstriction	Balanced approach to ventilation

superseded by focused assessment with sonography for trauma to detect free fluid; in general, this modality is preferable as it can also give an indication of fetal activity and heartbeat.

Radiation in pregnancy (Table 4.6)

Adverse effects are unlikely at less than 5–10 rads; most trauma patients are exposed to less than 3 rads.

- Use clinical judgement and shield the fetus as much as is possible during x-ray
- The relative risk (RR) of childhood cancers is highest in the first trimester (RR=3.19) and particularly high before 8 weeks of gestation (RR=4.6)

Trauma effect on the pregnancy

In early pregnancy the fetus is in a protected position in the pelvis. In later pregnancy the fetus is surrounded by amniotic fluid which cushions it but does not protect against penetrating trauma. The major risk to the fetus is through failure of the maternoplacental unit if the mother becomes shocked or hypoxic, or shearing injury.

> The most common injury to the fetus is hypoxia as a result of maternal hypovolaemia or damage to the uteroplacental apparatus

Placental abruption

- Separation of the placenta from the uterus
- Can cause major concealed haemorrhage (up to 2000 ml)

TABLE 4.6 Radiation dose to unshielded uterus (rads)	
Investigation	*Radiation dose to unshielded uterus (rads)*
Cervical spine x-ray	Undetectable
Anteroposterior (AP) chest x-ray	Up to 0.0043
Lumbar spine (AP)	Up to 4
Thoracic spine (AP)	<0.001
CT head	<0.05
CT thorax	Up to 0.6
CT upper abdomen	3.0–3.5
CT whole abdomen	2.8–4.6

- Disseminated intravascular coagulation
- Can jeopardize fetal placental blood flow
- Rarely there is amniotic fluid embolus
- Abruption has been reported in up to 50% of patients with major traumatic injuries, but can occur in up to 5% of relatively minor trauma cases
- Presentation can be delayed for 1–3 days

 Abruption can occur up to 72 h post trauma

- There is a risk of abruption from 12 weeks onwards but it characteristically occurs after 16 weeks of gestation

Symptoms
- Uterine contractions
- Vaginal bleeding
- Uterine tenderness
- Abdominal pain
- Abnormalities on fetal monitoring

However, these classical signs may be absent in nearly half of cases.

After 20 weeks' gestation external cardiotocography (CTG) monitoring can detect uterine contractions and is useful in assessing the uterine status. If there are less than 8 contractions per hour then there is considered to be a low risk of fetal/uterine injury. In general, monitoring is performed only when there is considered to be the chance of fetal viability (this may vary from institution to institution but is generally around 23 weeks). Before then obstetric management will not affect fetal survival. An approximate estimate of fetal age can be made using the simple technique shown in Figure 4.1.

After 24 weeks or where there is doubt commence monitoring as quickly as possible. Fetal tachycardia, loss of beat to beat variation, late decelerations and bradycardia (<120 bpm) should alert the team to a potential abruption. Normal monitoring for 4 h is highly reassuring. However, monitoring may be prudent for longer in high-risk mechanisms.

The normal fetal heart rate is 120–160 bpm

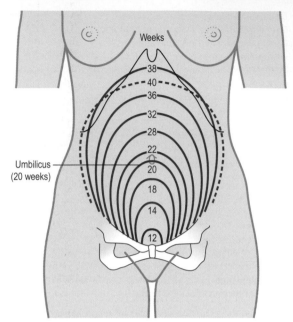

Figure 4.1 Uterine height and estimation of gestational age

Even in relatively minor trauma monitoring is required for a few hours. In more serious cases a minimum of 24-h monitoring is indicated. Ultrasound by an experienced obstetric sonographer is needed to recognize placental separation (however, caution is advised in the apparently negative scan!)

Classic signs of abruption
- Triad of tetanic/hypertonic contractions, abdominal pain and per vagina bleeding
- These signs are not infrequently absent!

Ruptured uterus
- Infrequent (less than 1%) event in major trauma but a potentially life-threatening condition
- Invariably associated with a major direct blow to the abdomen and often with a pelvic fracture

- The fetal mortality rate in such cases is near to 100% (those cases in which survival is reported had immediate surgery)

Penetrating trauma

This type of trauma carries a particularly high mortality rate for the fetus but less so for the mother (5%). For this reason, aim to deliver all viable pregnancies with penetrating trauma rapidly.

Premature labour

Premature labour occurs after trauma in one in ten pregnancies and early labour in one in four. For this reason, obstetric and neonatal teams need to be ready, and the equipment for delivery and neonatal resuscitation made available to all trauma patients in anticipation of a precipitous delivery.

Direct fetal injury

This is a relatively rare phenomenon as the fetus is effectively protected from shock by its surrounding amniotic fluid. However, skull fractures can be suffered as a result of pelvic trauma and these carry a high fetal mortality rate. Penetrating injuries may cause direct injury to any part of the fetus.

Burns

Treat as in the non-pregnant. However, aggressive fluid treatment so as to avoid maternal shock necessitates the input of specialists early. Also, caution should be taken regarding silver sulfadiazine cream as it may lead to kernicterus.

Pelvic trauma in pregnancy

Perhaps the most challenging condition is the pregnant woman with a major pelvic injury.

- Temporary pelvic slings (e.g. bedsheet or commercial pelvic sling) may buy a period of time and temporize the pelvic volume
- Major disruption puts the fetus at major risk as well as making normal vaginal delivery difficult

Each situation needs a balanced decision, taking into account gestational age, maternal status, fetal status and other injuries. Decisions are amongst the most complex in trauma and need to involve the combined expertise of the emergency, surgery, obstetrics, anaesthetic and critical care, neonatal and orthopaedic departments.

Post-mortem caesarean delivery

- Survival of the fetus is good if the interval between arrest and delivery is less than 5 min, but poor if longer than 25 min
- A gestational age of over 24 weeks is considered necessary (a simple guide is a fundus that reaches the umbilicus)
- Some authors would suggest that between 24 and 32 weeks attempts at internal cardiac massage should be made first to see if this works—if it does attempts at delivery may be delayed to try and improve survival of the very premature fetus

 The obstetric and neonatal team must be activated once a call has been received

Autotransfusion: antiD immunization

Autotransfusion is a risk in all cases; this includes the first trimester. Blood group and type must be determined in all cases, even in the most minor trauma. It is advisable (in line with local policy) to give antiD within 72 h to all Rhesus-negative women with abdominal trauma, even in what may be considered relatively minor injuries.

AntiD must be administered to all Rh-negative mothers within 72 h, including 'minor' abdominal trauma

Summary

- Give high flow oxygen to all pregnant trauma victims
- The airway is always at risk
- Relieve the caval pressure
- Give fluid before the apparent onset of shock
- Get early input from all teams
- The absence of fetal heart sounds is universally ominous for the fetus
- Don't forget antiD in the Rhesus-negative patient
- If the mother arrests deliver the baby
- Always be prepared for a precipitous delivery/caesarean

 The commonest cause of fetal death is maternal death

FURTHER READING

ACOG educational bulletin 1999 Obstetric aspects of trauma management. International Journal of Gynecology and Obstetrics 64:87–94

Drost T F, Rosemurgy A S, Sherman H F 1990 Major trauma in pregnant women: maternal/fetal outcome. Journal of Trauma 30:574–578

Morris J A, Rosenbower T J, Jurkovich G J et al 1996 Infant survival after caesarean section for trauma. Annals of Surgery 223:481–491

Shah K H, Simons R K 1998 Trauma in pregnancy; maternal and fetal outcomes. Journal of Trauma 45(1):83–86

CARE OF INFECTED AND IMMUNOCOMPROMISED PATIENTS

Background

The presence of infection or altered immunity may complicate the management of injured patients. The risks are twofold—those affecting patient care and outcome, and the potential risk to staff.

Patients at increased risk

Various medical and social backgrounds are implicated. Examples include

- Those with chronic medical and surgical conditions, including post-splenectomy patients
- Poor nutritional status, alcohol and substance abuse
- Malignancy
- Drug-induced immunosuppression, including steroids, particularly in post-transplant patients

History and examination

- Often the presence of a pre-existing risk will be offered by both the patient and previous medical records
- Signs of infection or altered immunity are sought during the secondary survey and include pyrexia, non-trauma-related tachypnoea or tachycardia, lymphadenopathy, splenomegaly, cellulitis and phlebitis
- When the patient's background is unknown be suspicious of the unexplained, the unusual and the unknown

Investigations

Further evidence may follow from blood tests and haematology (anaemia, absolute and differential white cell count), liver function tests (including serum albumin), erythrocyte sedimentation rate and C-reactive protein. Blood and tissue cultures may be necessary to assist in diagnosis and subsequent treatment. Imaging will initially involve common investigations such as chest x-ray but may require more sophisticated techniques at a later stage.

The risk to the patient

Clearly any increased risk is a result of the combination of the existing problem and the injury sustained. In practice, problems can arise from

- Reduced physiological reserve in the presence of injury
- Delayed and poor wound healing
- Exacerbation or progression of the pre-existing pathology
- Polypharmacy and antibiotic resistance
- Potential increased susceptibility to hospital-acquired infections

The risk to staff

This is the possibility of acquiring infection through direct contact, with body fluids, inhalation or inoculation—usually needlestick injury.

The real risk is that which is not known; this is minimized by preparation and adherence to some simple rules and common sense.

- Wear appropriate protective clothing at all times, particularly in respect to gloves
- With patients in extremis staff tend to neglect personal protective equipment in the rush to resuscitate the casualty; this should be avoided

 Always protect yourself

- Respect and adhere to local infection control and occupational health policies, particularly in respect to hepatitis B
- Take responsibility for cross infection; wash your hands between patients and use skin scrubs as supplied
- In the unlikely event of a needlestick injury, know and comply with the local policies for investigation and treatment

Ensure that all members of the trauma team wear appropriate personal protective equipment

Minimal personal protective equipment
Gloves
Impervious gown
Face mask
Goggles/visor
Lead apron

Patient management
The effect of infection or immunocompromise on the patient will
vary with the severity of the pre-existing condition(s) and the
trauma sustained. The principles of clinical care are

- Establish previous tetanus immunity—immunize or boost as
  necessary
- Ensure asplenic patients have had, or will receive, vaccines as per
  British National Formulary guidance
- Do not vaccinate chemotherapy patients without specialist
  advice
- Take all necessary samples for microbiology before giving
  prophylactic antibiotics. When completing specimen forms
  ensure that the medical history is sufficient to ensure proper
  interpretation by the laboratory
- Involve specialist help as necessary, particularly in respect of the
  ongoing management of underlying morbidity or the need for
  specialized products, e.g. irradiated blood products. Be prepared
  to measure and adjust blood levels of therapeutic agents
  according to microbiology advice
- Consider need for increased steroid dosage after injury
- Always interpret laboratory and radiology results in light of the
  history
- Reduce the risk to other patients. Liaise with nursing
  colleagues to ensure necessary precautions are taken in the
  management and placement of patients in the operating theatre
  and the wards

Summary
- Trauma patients frequently present with complicated medical
  and social backgrounds
- Infections such as hepatitis B, HIV and other forms of
  immunosuppression are not uncommon
- Be alert to the unusual and protect yourself at all times

TRAUMA CARE OF CONTAMINATED PATIENTS

Background

The threats of terrorism and industrial accidents have both increased the probability of having to deal with contaminated patients from chemical, biological, radiological or nuclear (CBRN) incidents. Injured CBRN patients would usually be expected to present in large numbers as part of a major incident. Planning and preparation for disaster entails a multi-agency response of which medical care of injured survivors is key component. It is a statutory requirement that any acute NHS Trust has a major incident plan which must include arrangements for decontamination of patients and appropriate protection for staff.

Definition of contamination

For our purposes this is the deliberate or accidental exposure to hazardous physical or biological material known to cause morbidity or death.

The contamination may be

- External: skin or clothing
- Internal: inhalation, ingestion (hand to mouth, or food and water), or through wound absorption

It is to be expected that in the context of trauma, contaminants are likely to be dispersed via conventional explosive devices causing blast injury.

Principles of dealing with contaminated casualties

The safety of staff is a priority. The degree of personal protective equipment must match the known or perceived threat. When a major incident has been declared pre-hospital many casualties will arrive already decontaminated. There will, however, always be patients who have bypassed this process. Trauma care, as always, follows the <C>ABC sequence, with the additional consideration that removal of clothing, decontamination and possible antidote administration become part of the resuscitation process.

The principles of treatment are

- Decontaminate and resuscitate in a dirty zone
- Transfer to clean zone(s) for ongoing definitive care

This is a one-way system in which the decontamination area is defined physically and policed by 'dirty' (outside) and 'clean' (inside) monitors who are responsible for staff safety.

Notes on specific threats

Chemical
This is the most likely threat following a terrorist incident. It is also possible following road, rail, aviation or industrial accident. Casualties will present with acute symptoms involving skin and respiratory systems. Specific antidotes may be available.

Biological
This may be a covert threat that only reveals itself following an incubation period. When dealing with patients following a documented suspicious incident that has occurred some time previously, always beware of the unknown, the unexplained or the unexpected.

Radiation
This could occur following a nuclear accident or as a consequence of a terrorist 'dirty bomb' (conventional explosive used to disseminate radioactive material). After exposure to ionizing radiation, life-threatening injuries can be treated prior to decontamination. Definitive trauma care ideally occurs early, as complications from radiation sickness will occur at 48 h to 2 weeks.

Nuclear
This would involve large scale casualties presenting with radiation and thermal injury. Comorbidity would lead to high mortality rates. When dealing with patients with minor injuries following an incident that has occurred some time previously, always beware of the unknown, the unexplained or the unexpected.

Summary
Effective care of the injured can only occur if you are safe. In respect of CBRN casualties preparation and planning is critical.

Locate, read, understand and, if necessary, question your local major incident plan!

Finally, a note of reassurance
Despite the sinister overtones of much of this material, it is a fact that basic infection control personal protective equipment will afford considerable or complete protection for many of the possible hazards. This means a theatre scrub suit, disposable apron, double gloves, mask with visor and head cover.

FURTHER READING

Web Sites Health Protection Agency (HPA) www.hpa.org.uk/emergency/
CBRNhtm CBRN incidents; clinical management and health protection
Department of Health (DOH) www.dh.gov.uk NHS emergency planning
guide 2005
UK resilience (a service of the cabinet office) January 2007 www.
ukresilience.info/emergencies/cbrn.shtm

CHAPTER 5

MECHANISM OF INJURY

OVERVIEW OF TRAUMA EPIDEMIOLOGY

Incidence of trauma

In the developed world, in those under 40 years old, *injury* is the commonest cause of death. Trauma is the third most common cause of death across all age groups.

Regional variation

Injury rates vary geographically. In developing countries standards of living are lower and infection is the leading important cause of death: however, injury prevention strategies and effective trauma systems are less developed so trauma remains the second commonest cause.

Gender

Trauma is generally associated with some form of risk-taking behaviour. It is not therefore surprising that young men are over-represented in the injury statistics.

Age

Risk-taking behaviour is inversely correlated with age, and the incidence of injury peaks in the third decade of life. However, there is a second peak in later life when musculoskeletal failure results in injury after activities that are less vigorous.

WHY?

Haddon matrix

A common way of analysing cause of injury is the *Haddon matrix*. This cross references the host, agent and environmental factors with pre-event, event and post-event factors. Host factors include age, gender and comorbidity; the agent may be a motor vehicle or a work tool; environmental factors may be the road, the ambient temperature or the level of lighting. Combinations of these factors may be present and may interact with the injury before, during and after the event (Table 5.1).

Medical care is part of the post-event phase, and relates to the physical and social aspects of the environment which interacts with the patient after injury.

Injury may be accidental (in the sense that the injured person had no intent to injure themselves), inflicted by others or self-inflicted. In some parts of the world, in the young male population, suicide may be a more common cause of death than accidental injury.

TABLE 5.1 The Haddon matrix			
P	*Factor*		
H	Host	Agent	Environment
A	Pre-event		
S	Event		
E	Post-event		

Interpersonal violence can result in either blunt or penetrating injury, with the proportion of each dependent upon the availability of weapons.

WHEN?

Time of day
Trauma occurs most commonly in leisure time, thus evenings are a more common time for presentation than in the morning hours.

Day of week
Although work-related injury represents a significant proportion of the burden of injury, risk-taking behaviour contributed to by drug and alcohol use play a much more significant role. Injury rates are therefore higher on typical weekend periods. In the Western world this is commonly on Friday evening, Saturday and Sunday.

Month of year
In countries with severe climates, recreational activities are severely restricted during winter. Conversely, during summer recreational activities increase and therefore injury rates are increased. In countries with more even climates there is no such variation.

WHERE?

Road traffic-related injury remains a significant cause of severe trauma in most parts of the developed and developing world, and hence much severe trauma occurs at the roadside. Falls represent the most common cause of injury, usually at a less severe level, and these occur in or around the home. Interpersonal violence usually occurs at locations where people gather, such as shows and clubs.

Summary

Trauma is a cause of both immediately life-threatening and less severe presentations for healthcare in every part of the world. In general it is most likely to be

- Young men
- After hours
- Blunt trauma

MOTOR VEHICLE COLLISIONS

Background

Motor vehicle collisions (MVC) are the third most common cause of death worldwide, causing more than 1 million deaths and 38 million injuries each year. This is projected to increase substantially over the next few decades, as the number of vehicles on the roads continues to increase, especially in developing countries.

Statistics

In the USA in 2002

- There were 42 815 fatalities and more than 5 million injuries related to MVCs
- More than 356 000 individuals suffered incapacitating injuries requiring hospitalization
- Americans have a one in three chance of being involved in a severe MVC in their lifetime
- Drivers are four times more likely to be involved in a car accident if operating a cell phone

Pre-hospital information

Information from emergency personnel about the MVC can aid in evaluating the patient.

- The estimated speed of all vehicles involved
- Was it a head-on, side, or rear impact?
- Did the vehicle roll over?
- Were the occupants wearing seatbelts?
- Were they ejected?
- Did the car have airbags that deployed?
- How long did extrication take?
- The type of vehicle and the extent of damage to it

Injury mechanisms

The mechanism of the MVC can suggest particular injury patterns (Table 5.2).

TABLE 5.2 Suspected injuries by mechanism of motor vehicle collision

Mechanisms of injury	Suspected injuries
Frontal	Head — subdural haemorrhage — facial trauma Neck — cervical spine fracture Chest — myocardial contusion — pneumothorax — rib fractures — pulmonary contusion — traumatic aortic disruption — tracheal disruption Abdomen — spleen or liver injury — bucket handle injuries to mesentery Extremities — posterior knee or hip dislocation

Side	Neck
	— cervical spine fracture
	Chest
	— rib fractures/flail chest
	— pneumothorax
	— diaphragmatic rupture
	— traumatic aortic disruption
	Abdomen
	— liver or spleen injury
	   depending on relationship of passenger to site of impact
	— pelvic fractures
	Extremities
	— long bone fractures
	   depending of relationship of passenger to site of impact

Rear	Neck — whiplash
Rollover	Variable and multifactorial — normally less then suspected owing to dispersion of energy over entire vehicle Ejection? Wearing safety devices?
Ejection	No predictable pattern Greater risk of all injuries

Essentials

- Restrained passengers
  - risk of injuries from lap seatbelt (seatbelt sign) to the aorta, intestine and carotid artery
- Unrestrained passengers
  - 50% will have some level of traumatic brain injury
  - more likely to have been in back seat or in a commercial vehicle (i.e. taxi)
  - unrestrained passengers in the back seat increase mortality rates of those in the front seats
- Rollover
  - because of varying forces there is no predictable injury pattern
- Ejections
  - four times more likely to require admission to hospital because of injuries
  - fivefold increase in injury severity score
  - three times more likely to have associated head trauma
  - increased risk for hypothermia and exposure-related injuries
- Effects of safety devices
  - 11% decreased mortality from proper airbag use
  - 41% decreased mortality from proper seatbelt use
  - 69% decreased mortality from proper use of child safety seats
- Pitfalls
  - seat belt injury
    abrasion/contusion running from shoulder to contralateral hip
    traumatic aorta or pulmonary artery rupture
    tracheal disruption requires bronchoscopy
    bucket handle tears in the mesentery
  - carotid artery dissection
    high association with other cervical spine injuries
    present with either focal neurological defect or seizure
    angiography for diagnosis

TABLE 5.3 Mortality rate by collision type

Motor vehicle collision type	Mortality rate (%)
Frontal	50–60
Side	20–35
Rear	3–5
Rollover	8–15

MOTORCYCLE COLLISIONS

Background

Worldwide, motorcycles and bicycles are used more commonly than any other vehicles for transportation. Motorcycles are less stable and less visible than cars, and have high performance capabilities. For these and other reasons, motorcycles are more likely than cars to be involved in crashes. When involved in a crash, owing to the lack of protection conferred from the motorcycle (compared to an enclosed vehicle), riders are more likely to be injured or killed.

- Per mile travelled, the number of deaths on motorcycles is about 16 times the number in cars
- Helmets have been shown to be effective in preventing motorcycle deaths and brain injuries
- Death rates from head injuries are twice as high among non-helmeted compared to motorcyclists wearing helmets
- A motorcyclist is three times as likely to be injured
- A quarter of all accidents involve only the motorcyclist
- Weather or road defects are the cause in less than 2% of crashes
- The median pre-crash speed was 29.8 mph (50 kph)
- One of every thousand crashes takes place at a speed of approximately 86 mph (143 kph)

Injuries

Injuries sustained in motorcycle collisions are shown in Table 5.4.

Essentials

- Factors contributing to motorcycle collisions
  — male
  — age <25 years
  — inexperience
  — alcohol
  — curves in road
  — riding during peak hours
  — not being licensed to ride a motorcycle
  — new motorcycle
    20% of accidents occur during the first or second time riding the motorcycle
- Prevention
  — motorcyclist safety programs can reduce motorcycle collisions by upwards of 69%
  — wearing a helmet reduces the likelihood of fatality by 29–35%
  — fatality rates are twice as high in states without mandatory helmet laws

TABLE 5.4 Suspected injuries by area of body in motorcycle collisions

Area	Suspected injuries
Head	Head injury is a leading cause of death in motorcycle crashes Concussion Closed head injury Coup-contrecoup Diffuse axonal injury Intracranial haemorrhage Subdural haematoma Facial trauma
Neck	Whiplash Cervical spine fracture
Chest	Myocardial contusion Pneumothorax Rib fractures/flail chest Pulmonary contusion Traumatic aortic disruption Tracheal disruption Thoracic spine fracture
Abdomen	Spleen or liver injury Pancreas injury Handlebar injury in children Pelvic fractures
Extremities	Posterior cruciate ligament tear Popliteal artery injury Long bone fractures Most commonly lower legs Tibia and fibula most common

— nearly half of fatally injured motorcyclists were not wearing helmets
— helmet use has clearly been shown to lower healthcare costs

AUTO VS. PEDESTRIAN

Background

Thousands of pedestrians are killed each year. Collectively in the past 30 years, nearly 200 000 pedestrians have died in all motor vehicle crashes in the USA. Alcohol is a major contributor to these injuries.

- 30% of pedestrians and 20% of drivers are under the influence of alcohol

Auto vs. pedestrian crashes produce complicated but distinctive injury patterns that must be considered when evaluating these patients. The practitioner is often faced with identifying and caring for multiply injured patients with closed head injuries, intra-abdominal, intrathoracic and orthopaedic injuries.

Essentials
- Children and the elderly are at high risk of being run over
- People who have taken drugs or alcohol are at high risk of being run over
- The injury pattern is a direct consequence of body size (children vs. adults) and vehicle type (van, sports utility vehicle (SUV) or passenger vehicle)
- Approximately 75% of patients have extremity injuries
- Do not be distracted by extremity fractures; instead focus on the injuries that are potentially life-threatening
- Most pedestrian fatalities occur at night, during the weekends and at non-intersection locations

Injury patterns associated with auto vs. pedestrian accidents
With accidents that involve passenger cars

- Adult injury classically involves three separate impacts
  — initial impact with the lower extremities, as the front of the braking vehicle lowers during rapid deceleration (Fig. 5.1)
  — second impact as the casualty is thrown on the hood of the vehicle, striking their thorax and head
  — third impact as the casualty is thrown to the ground, again striking their head
- Paediatric injury is variable and less predictable than adults
  — children are often thrown away from the vehicle or run over
  — injuries include chest, abdomen, closed head injuries and multisystem injuries (Fig. 5.2)

  With accidents involving light trucks (SUVs) and vans
- The injury pattern can be very different from that of passenger cars. These vehicles have higher bumpers and their higher point of impact more commonly results in chest and abdominal injuries (Fig. 5.3)

Do not be distracted by extremity wounds. Focus on potentially life-threatening injuries

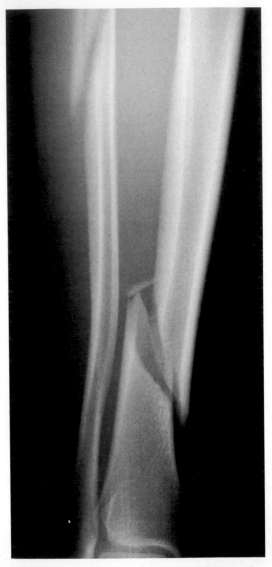

Figure 5.1 Classic lower extremity injury (tibia and fibula fractures) in an adult pedestrian that was struck

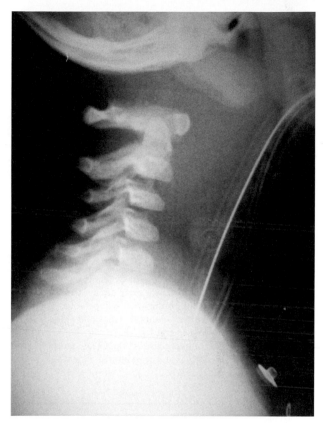

Figure 5.2 Atlanto-occipital dissociation in a child that was fatally struck by a motor vehicle

Remember:

- Patients with blunt trauma can have multiple injuries that require different surgical subspecialty expertise for optimal management. Resources take time to mobilize so it is important to plan ahead

 BEWARE
Occult vascular injuries can be elusive; consider popliteal and cerebrovascular injuries

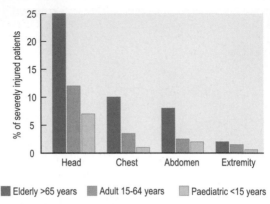

Figure 5.3 Distribution of injury following pedestrian accidents

Pitfalls

- Do not get distracted and focus on the extremity injuries that are often associated with auto vs. pedestrian accidents
- Neurological and vascular examination is imperative; do not forget about vertebral artery, popliteal artery and other less obvious but high morbidity injuries
- Even a single episode of hypotension can increase morbidity and mortality rates, especially in the head-injured patient
- Mobilize your resources early

FALLS

Background
Unintentional falls account for a substantial number of deaths and are the leading cause of non-fatal injuries.

 15 000 people die from falls in the USA annually

Falls are the leading cause of injury-related death in people over the age of 65 years and are one of the biggest threats to independent living in this population. In children younger than 14 years, falls are the number one cause of non-fatal injury.

Injuries obtained after falls from height can be extensive, with highly variable injury patterns. However, there are some well recognized injury patterns associated with 'axial load type falls' in which the patient lands upright or in a seated position.

Essentials
- Low height falls in children, falls in the elderly, and falls from height can all result in high morbidity and mortality rates
- The LD50 is the height from which a fall will result in death in 50% of the casualties
- For falls from height the LD50 is approximately 8–10 m (25–30 feet) or three stories
- Falls from standing or low heights can still result in significant morbidity and life-threatening injury
- Do not be distracted by extremity fractures; instead focus on the *associated injuries* that are potentially life-threatening
- The death rate *doubles* in falls greater than 5 m (15 feet)
- Falls in the elderly are often associated with concurrent medical events, e.g. myocardial infarct, transient ischaemic attack

Death and injury are primarily dependent upon

- Height of the fall
- Composition of the landing surface
- Age of the patient
- If the fall was slowed or broken by an intervening object
- Position in which the patient landed

Injury patterns (Fig. 5.6)
- Adult falls from low heights (standing, bed, stairs)
  — may result in single system, life-threatening injury (fatal closed head injuries can result from falls from low heights)
  — aside from closed head injury, cervical spine, soft tissue, orthopaedic and chest wall injuries are common
  — *many patients in an ageing patient population are on anticoagulants*
- Adult falls from height
  — upright landings can result in multiple injuries, but classically include
  calcaneal and lower extremity injuries (Fig. 5.4)
  vertical shear injuries of the pelvis
  fractures of the thoracic and lumbar spines
  other deceleration injuries, including transection of the aorta (at aortic root or ligamentum arteriosum) or avulsion of the renal pedicle (Fig. 5.5)

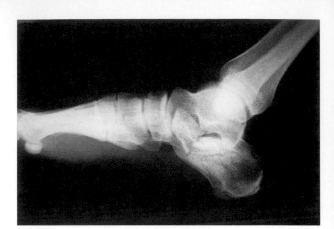

Figure 5.4 Calcaneal fracture sustained during an axial load upright landing from a fall

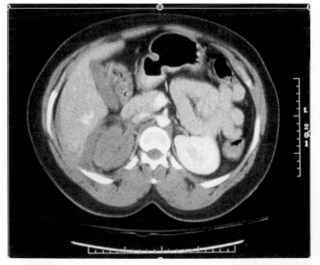

Figure 5.5 Vertical shear injury of renal pedicle with absence of perfusion of the patient's right kidney

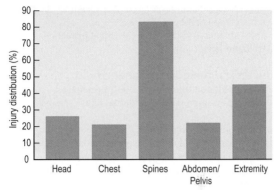

Figure 5.6 Distribution of injury following falls from height in the adult patient

Geriatric falls

- Falls in this population constitute a major health problem, resulting in up to 7 million injuries per year
- The 6-month mortality rate of elderly patients who sustain a hip fracture during a fall is 25%, with the 1-year mortality rate approaching 50%
- One-third of the elderly who live at home and up to 50 % of elderly people living in nursing homes sustain falls
- 25% sustain serious injury
- Concurrent medical emergencies that triggered the fall may complicate management

Paediatric falls

- Paediatric falls result in approximately 100–150 deaths annually in the USA
  — they occur secondary to falls from windows, fire escapes, balconies or roofs
  — falls lead to extremity, thoracic and closed head injuries
  — younger children have disproportionately large heads and lack the ability to right themselves, therefore often landing head first
- Paediatric falls from low heights (less than 5 m; 15 feet)
  — although counterintuitive, low height falls (e.g. climbing frames, 'monkey bars') cause many injuries

— intra-abdominal injury is as common from low height falls as it is from falls over 5 m (15 feet)
— approximately 14% of children sustain intracranial injury from low height falls

Resuscitation/immediate management

- Initial resuscitation follows <C>ABC principles
- No matter how impressive the external injuries, remember the <C>ABCs
- Identify life-threatening injuries
- In cases of closed head injury, avoid secondary insults including even transient episodes of hypoxia or hypotension
- In elderly patients think about comorbidity and be prepared to reverse anticoagulation

> Try to identify a cause for the fall, especially in the elderly population; often these events have cardiovascular or neurovascular precipitants

> Be alert for classic axial load injury patterns related to falls from height:
> - Association of calcaneal fracture
> - With lower extremity fracture (as high as 50%)
> - With lumbar spine fracture (as high as 15%)

Pitfalls

- Look objectively at the entire picture; often the immediate threat to life is the medical cause of the fall, not the result of the fall
- Because many elderly patients are already prone to falling, be wary of splints, braces and casts that may exacerbate an existing fall risk
- Many older patients are taking anticoagulants and are thus at increased risk for uncontrolled intracranial or other haemorrhage
- Many elderly patients are osteopenic and are therefore at increased risk of fractures from falls
- Older patients may be on chronotropic agents which may prevent them from becoming tachycardic
- Inadequate pain control (i.e. failing to place an epidural for chest trauma) can result in great morbidity

- Falls in infants should be carefully screened for abuse; rolling off an elevated surface or bed is inconsistent with age less than 6 months

> Often, injuries which are not identified on the initial surveys don't become apparent until the tertiary survey, which can be hours or days later. These injuries may remain elusive until the patient can localize pain

Prevention

> Help prevent future injuries; discuss environmental risk factors of falls (removal of obstacles, placement of throw rugs and hazards of steep steps) with your elderly patients

IMPALEMENT

 Do not be distracted by the impalement
Treat the life-threatening injuries

A wide variety of impaling objects and associated injuries have been reported but, unlike knife wounds that generally involve cutting of soft tissue localized to the path of the blade, major impalement often involves a combination of penetrating and blunt injury.

All manifestations of major blunt organ injury can occur, and associated skin lacerations are frequently irregularly shaped, ragged and dirty.

The impaling object may be irregular in shape and size and, if the object is large and blunt, the considerable force required to pierce the body is also transmitted bluntly to local structures.

- A large, blunt impaling object can push aside organs such as the lung or bowel
- The impaling object may exert compression to local structures and major vessels, inhibiting exsanguination or visceral contamination in some cases
- The impaling object drives dirty foreign material into contact with damaged or ischaemic tissue

- For patient transport the object should be shortened then immobilized to the skin to prevent secondary injury or accidental dislodgement

> Impaling objects must only be removed when vascular control has been obtained in an operating environment

Pitfalls
- Expect a combination of penetrating and blunt injuries from an impaling object
- Impalement wounds are generally dirty, requiring meticulous debridement
- Other serious injuries may be overshadowed by the impalement
- The impaling object should be shortened and immobilized prior to patient transport
- Only remove impaling objects with vascular control in an operating environment to avoid exsanguination

KNIVES

Background
Knives are available, concealable and lethal, and the wide variety of types is reflected in the wide variety of the wounds they cause. In all but the most superficial lacerations it is difficult to determine the severity and anatomical extent of injury accurately on the basis of a skin wound and an inferred mechanism of injury.

It is not enough to simply diagnose injury; potentially serious occult injuries must be excluded by thorough examination and appropriate diagnostic procedures.

Wounds
Commonly used weapons are kitchen knives, pocket knives, flick knives and a range of hunting or military weapons. In general

- Cutting blades leave a clean apex to a skin wound
- Serrated blades leave a ragged edge
- Double-edged blades leave a fusiform wound
- Single-edged blades may cause a boat-shaped wound

Stretch in the skin can make an entry wound smaller than the width of the blade once it is removed from the patient.

Twisting or rocking of the blade against the fulcrum of the skin can cause extensive internal damage at the time of the initial incident or during transport if the blade is in situ but unsupported.

Estimation of the depth and direction of penetration
by examination of the blade and surface wound
characteristics may be unreliable for the following
reasons
- Owing to the position of the patient's body at the time
  of injury
- The compressive effect of the impact causing injury
  deeper than the depth of the blade

Injury

All penetrating wounds of the head, neck, torso or extremities
proximal to the elbows or knees warrant trauma team activation as
they have potential to cause major occult injury to vessels, nerves
and soft tissues.

 Always examine the back, perineum, groins and axillas

Don't poke holes

Head and neck

Prime structures of concern are vessels, nerves and tubes (the
nasopharynx, trachea and oesophagus).

- Severe and potentially life-threatening injuries may initially be
  occult but should be immediately excluded by clinical assessment
  and appropriate diagnostic tests
- Skull or bony penetration may result in broken blade fragments
  which are not apparent on clinical examination
- The skull may be penetrated by a combination of the cutting
  point and the blunt force of impact
- A stabbing blade can reach any structure in the neck depending
  on the zone of penetration and trajectory
- Transverse slashing incisions of the front of the neck (cut-throat)
  pierce the skin, platysma, strap muscles, thyroid, trachea and
  then the large vessels

Torso

In the thorax, piercing injuries to the lungs and heart are evidenced
by haemothorax, pneumothorax, air leak or cardiac tamponade.

- Lacerations of the diaphragm are difficult to exclude without visual inspection unless herniation of abdominal contents has already occurred
- Abdominal structures are exposed to injury if the blade has traversed the thorax below the nipple line or if a particularly long blade such as a long pointed kitchen knife has been used
- The abdominal structures at greatest risk in a thoracic stab are the liver, stomach, transverse colon, small bowel, duodenum, spleen and pancreas
- Most self-inflicted knife stab injuries are on the right side
- Beware stab wounds above the buttock crease; they can traverse the pelvis and injure bowel

 Peritoneal breach *must* be excluded if the anterior fascia of the abdominal wall is breached

Extremities

Limb loss is usually the result of devastating vascular injury although long-term deficits are usually the result of nerve injury. The peripheral vascular tree is relatively protected from blunt injury by the ability of vessels to stretch and bend, but they are exposed to injury by a sharp blade.

- Transection of an artery may be followed by vascular spasm which can be intense enough to close the vessel lumen
- Tangential or ragged lacerations can obliterate this protective spasm, leading to profuse ongoing bleeding
- Bony impact can cause blade breakage and retention of fragments which can be missed on physical examination
- Capsular penetration should be excluded from any stab wound around a joint

Pitfalls

- Major damage may be inflicted through a small wound
- Estimations of wound depth and trajectory from the appearance of the skin wound are unreliable
- Knives remaining in situ should be supported and immobilized until surgical removal
- A knife in the torso may traverse the diaphragm
- Abdominal wall breach means peritoneal breach until proven otherwise

- Knife tips can break off when they hit bone. Plain radiography will show them

SHOOTINGS

Background

- Gunshot wounds impact greatly on healthcare and the criminal justice system
- There is a positive correlation between homicide rates and availability of guns in developed nations
- The level of gun ownership worldwide is directly related to murder and suicide rates, and specifically to the level of death by gunfire
- Handguns account for more than two-thirds of all firearm-related deaths each year
- A gun kept in the home is 22 times more likely to be used in a homicide, suicide or unintentional shooting than in self-defence
- Over 57% of all suicides are committed with a firearm

Essentials

- As of 1994, 44 million Americans owned more than 192 million firearms, of which 65 million were handguns
- At the end of 2001, in England and Wales there were 301 000 firearms (75% rifles) and 1 307 576 shotguns registered
- In 1998, handguns murdered 11 789 people in the USA, 373 in Germany, 151 in Canada, 54 in England and Wales, and 19 people in Japan
- The number of non-fatal injuries is considerable, with over 200 000 per year in the USA
- Despite strict legislation banning the ownership and use of guns in the UK, the number of gun-related offences increased from 9502 in 1989 to 24 094 in 2004; the number of injuries from firearms increased from 2164 to 4762 during the same time period

Anatomy of firearms

Handguns

- Handguns are compact weapons initially designed for self-defence
- Most handguns produce 'low velocity' projectiles (<1100 feet/s)
- They are 'concealable' and this is a part of the legal definition of a handgun

- Handguns are designed to fire multiple shots; the most common are revolvers and semiautomatic pistols
- Revolvers are limited to six shots, are less expensive and more accurate
- Semiautomatic pistols use recoil to eject the fired cartridge and are more conducive to firing multiple shots, with most carrying 15–19 rounds
- Semiautomatic versions of submachine guns (such as the Uzi) are classified as handguns because of their concealability

Rifles

- Rifles differ from handguns in the length of the barrel and the presence of a butt stock
- Rifling or grooves inside the barrel improve the accuracy
- Rifles are more accurate and shoot more powerful cartridges than handguns
- Rifles can produce projectiles with high velocities (up to and exceeding 3000 feet/s)
- Military rifles are semiautomatic or automatic, holding 5–50 rounds

Shotguns

- Shotguns have a similar external appearance to rifles, but do not have rifling inside the barrel
- A shotgun shell may contain one large projectile (a slug), a few pellets of large shot, or many tiny pellets
- Shotguns have a minimal capacity to wound humans at distances greater than 15 m, but blasts at close range (less than 1.5 m; 4 feet) are fatal in 85% of cases

Ballistics

- Ballistics refers to the science of the travel of a bullet in flight: down the barrel, through the air and through a target
- The longer the barrel (to a point), the greater the acceleration
- Kinetic energy (KE) delivered to a target can be calculated by the formula:

$$KE = \frac{1}{2} MV^2$$

where V = velocity in feet/s and M (mass) is given in pounds, derived from the weight of the bullet × acceleration of gravity
- Bullets do not typically follow a straight line; they are affected by rotational forces of yaw, precession and nutation, as seen in Fig. 5.7
- Terminal ballistics is the final complicated motion that occurs when a bullet strikes its target

Yaw

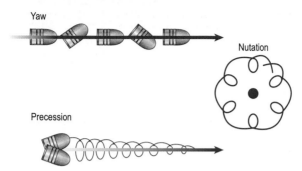

Nutation

Precession

Figure 5.7 Rotational forces that affect a bullet in flight include yaw, precession and nutation

- The KE from the bullet is transmitted to the target (tissues of the body); multiple factors such as velocity, bullet characteristics, type of tissue, and direction and distance of travel will influence the extent and type of injury
- Bullets can produce tissue damage in three ways
  - laceration and crushing: low-velocity bullets (in handguns) do virtually all of their damage via crushing
  - cavitation: this is significant with high-velocity projectiles. A 'permanent' cavity is caused by the path of the bullet itself, and a 'temporary' cavity is formed by stretching of the tissues (Fig. 5.8)
  - shock waves travel ahead and to the sides, and can approach up to 200 atmospheres of pressure with high-velocity wounds
- The distance of the target from the muzzle plays a large role in wounding capacity, especially for shotguns (Fig. 5.9)
- Bullet design is important in wounding potential
- Bullets that tumble, expand and fragment cause more damage as greater amounts of KE are transmitted to the tissues
- The Hague Convention of 1899 forbade the use of expanding deformable bullets in wartime. Therefore, military bullets have full metal jackets around the lead core to limit fragmentation and expansion (Fig. 5.10)
- The type of tissue affects wounding potential—the higher the specific gravity of the tissue, the greater the damage
- Liver, spleen and brain have no elasticity and are easily injured. Fluid-filled organs (bladder, heart, bowel and great vessels) can burst because of pressure waves generated

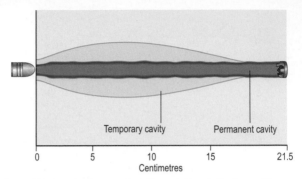

Figure 5.8 Example of a wound profile caused by a bullet from a 38 special (a common police gun). This is a low-velocity projectile travelling at 903 feet/s. (Redrawn with permission of Martin Fackler, COL, MC, USA (Ret.) www.FirearmsTactical.com 12 January 2007)

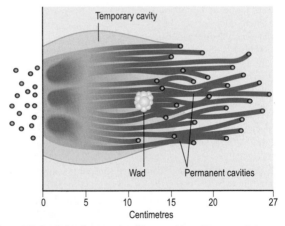

Figure 5.9 Example of a wound profile caused by a 12-gauge shotgun (close range) using 27 pellet no. 4 buck at 1350 feet/s. Note the extensive permanent cavities and the presence of the wadding in the wound. (Redrawn with permission of Martin Fackler, COL, MC, USA (Ret.) www. FirearmsTactical.com 12 January 2007)

- A bullet striking bone can cause fragmentation and secondary missiles that can cause additional damage
- Examples of wounding patterns for selected types of weapons are depicted in Figures 5.8–5.11

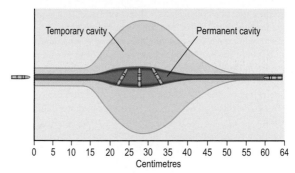

Figure 5.10 Example of a classic wound profile caused by a full metal jacket military bullet (a NATO 7.62 mm travelling at a high velocity of 2730 feet/s). Note that this modern jacketed non-fragmenting/ non-expanding bullet travels a great distance before it starts to tumble. (Redrawn with permission of Martin Fackler, COL, MC, USA (Ret.) www. FirearmsTactical.com 12 January 2007)

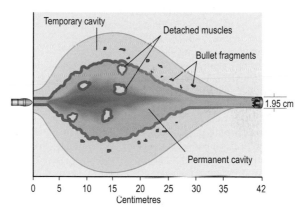

Figure 5.11 This wound profile is caused by a softpoint Winchester .30-06 150 gr with a velocity of 2923 feet/s. This bullet can be used in civilian hunting rifles. Note the extensive damage, with a large permanent cavity caused by expansion and fragmentation of the bullet. (Redrawn with permission of Martin Fackler, COL, MC, USA (Ret.) www.FirearmsTactical. com 12 January 2007)

Essentials of gunshot wound management

- Initial treatment of victims of gunshot wounds should be as for any trauma patient, with careful attention to the <C>ABCs

- Bleeding must be controlled by direct pressure, tourniquets, haemostatic dressings or prompt surgical intervention
- *Completely expose and examine the entire patient as additional wounds may be found (look in skin folds, axillae, genitalia, between buttocks, under hair, etc.)*
- Record the location, size and shape of all wounds made by a penetrating profile. Do not speculate on direction of fire or entrance/exit wound details unless you are in fact a ballistics expert
- The number of wounds and the number of retained bullets should add up to an even number. If not, an exhaustive search should be made for the missing hole or bullet. Remember, some patients may be repeat victims and have retained bullet(s) from a previous injury
- Remember, bullets do not respect tissue planes and may have traversed more than one body cavity
- X-rays (anteroposterior and lateral) are essential adjuncts to visualize retained bullets or fragments and can aid in determining the path of the bullet. Place radio-opaque markers (paper clips) on all penetrating wounds
- CT scans are useful adjuncts in patients who are haemodynamically stable to help identify potential intra-abdominal and intrathoracic injuries
- If a bullet or fragment enters a vascular space it can migrate
- Maintain a high index of suspicion for vascular injury and have a low threshold for angiography
- The best approach to wound care is conservative (irrigation and dressing often suffice)
- Remember tetanus prophylaxis
- Give antibiotics if indicated (recommended for high-velocity, shotgun, intra-articular and disruptive injuries)
- Judicious debridement of devitalized tissues is required when extensive tissue disruption is apparent. As viability of tissue can be difficult to determine, leave the wound open and continually re-evaluate during the first 48 h

 Treat the wound not the weapon

EXPLOSIONS

Background

Explosions predictably cause multiple casualties with complex combined injuries. The explosion may be accidental, for example from heating and motor fuels, fertilizers and paints. However, planning for casualties of an explosion must involve consideration of the terrorist improvised explosive device (IED). Military traumatologists must be prepared to deal with IEDs, landmines (vehicle and antipersonnel), ordnance (grenades, artillery rounds, mortar shells) and airborne munitions (bombs, cluster bombs and fuel–air explosives).

Mechanisms of injury

A populist classification is to describe four types of 'blast injury'

- *Primary*: injury from the overpressure from the blast wave
- *Secondary*: penetrating fragments of the explosive casing and destroyed items near the explosion
- *Tertiary*: blunt injury from displacement (thrown by the 'blast wind') or crushed under collapsing structures
- *Quaternary*: burns and inhalation injury (hot gases and combustion products)

This is a confusing classification for those unfamiliar with these injuries. A simpler and more functional classification that uses clear descriptive terms follows

- *Blast wave*: air compressed by the expanding sphere of hot gases forms a front of *overpressure*. Air in the middle ear and gut is compressed and heated. It then re-expands, leading to perforation. 'Spalling' occurs at air–tissue interfaces, leading to intra-alveolar haemorrhage (*blast lung*)
- *Blast wind*: this is the whoosh of air behind the blast wave that produces 'knock down' blunt trauma and traumatic avulsive amputations. It also carries fragments of 'street furniture', namely stones, splinters and glass that act as missiles
- *Fragmentation*: these are *primary* when they arise from the bomb casing and *secondary* when they are packed around the explosive (e.g. ballbearings, notched wire, nails)
- *Burns*: characteristically superficial, but deep burns are also possible
- *Crush*: if the building collapses

- *Psychological*: the principal aim of the terrorist is to change behaviour by inducing fear

These mechanisms can occur independently, but they can and usually do occur in combinations that complicate the management of each. *The commonest injuries seen following an explosion are from fragments.* The relationships between these mechanisms must be appreciated to organize the approach to victims of an explosion and avoid pitfalls that can lead to poor outcome. In general, the nature and severity of these injuries is predicted by the distance from the epicentre of the explosion (Fig. 5.12).

Terrorist bombs
All explosions can include fragments of surrounding items that are destroyed, including bone and tissue from victims. Human tissue as a missile is a major consideration in suicide bombings.

Terrorist IEDs intentionally use multiple small items to increase the number of fragments generated and maximize the number of victims. These can include nuts, bolts, nails and glass. Infectious agents and chemical warfare agents are a theoretical threat, but there is a likelihood that an explosion would destroy the chemical or infectious agent: non-explosive delivery systems are, however, feasible. Radiation contamination is also feasible by means of a 'dirty bomb'.

Terrorists often choose highly populated areas and enclosed spaces to maximize the impact of the blast wave. Research has identified a statistically higher injury severity and poorer outcome

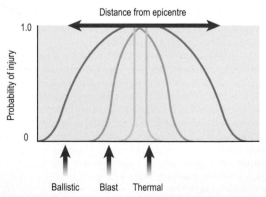

Figure 5.12 Probability of injury as a function of distance from epicentre of blast

with explosions in confined spaces (bus bombs compared to open air bombs in Israel).

Terrorists characteristically use a second (potentially larger) bomb after the first draws rescuers and onlookers. It is essential that the scene is cleared of secondary devices as the highest priority.

Mines

Large mines may overturn tanks or vehicles and cause injuries consistent with other explosive devices.

Most antipersonnel mines are designed to incapacitate rather than kill, as a wounded casualty consumes more of the enemy's resources than a dead casualty. There are exceptions, such as the bounding antipersonnel mine where a small charge kicks the mine out of the ground to chest height before the main charge detonates.

Typically, antipersonnel mines are triggered when stood on: the blast may remove the distal lower limb and the upward force raises tissue planes, causing central destruction along the bone and depositing debris higher than the external injury indicates (Fig. 5.13). Mine wounds of the limbs must be debrided thoroughly, and often demand a formal amputation with the flaps left open for delayed closure.

The perineum should be evaluated in lower extremity mine wounds to ensure that there are no small fragment wounds that penetrate the rectum, pelvis or abdomen.

Evaluation and treatment

Blast injury

- Penetrating, blunt and burn injuries are resusciated according to <C>ABC priorities
- Suspect and seek blast overpressure injuries

- In the open, the likelihood of blast injury is directly proportional to the distance from the explosion
- In enclosed spaces, the blast wave is reflected from solid surfaces and is enhanced. Different victims in the same room will have a different blast load
- Overpressure injuries generate much discussion, but with the exception of some military 'enhanced blast' weapons they usually form a minority of the injuries in patients *who survive*
- These injuries should be suspected and sought, especially if the patient was in an enclosed space, or has flash burns (these indicate proximity to the point of explosion)

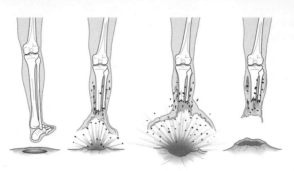

Figure 5.13 Mine injury to the lower extremity (Redrawn with permission of Martin Fackler, COL, MC, USA (Ret.) www.FirearmsTactical.com 12 January 2007)

- Abdominal visceral injury may not manifest for several days, so those who are unconscious should be evaluated frequently for fever, changes in clinical findings on abdominal examination, or new fluid collection on ultrasound or CT
- Those who otherwise have no injury and would be released should be instructed to return if they experience symptoms of progressive dyspnoea or abdominal visceral injury
- A ruptured tympanic membrane has been used to indicate exposure to a significant blast load, but it is a poor predictor of patients who progress to develop blast lung
- Following blast, animal model research identifies temporary apnoea and/or cardiac arrest that is reversible in the presence of no other major structural injury or catastrophic blood loss (e.g. limb loss)

Pitfalls in managing explosive injury

- Forgetting to evaluate and treat by <C>ABC priority
- Distraction from serious occult injury by obvious large soft tissue wounds
- Failure to control haemorrhage from large soft tissue wounds
- Inadequate debridement of debris and dead tissue along blast paths in tissue planes
- Missing intracavity wounds and large vessel injury caused by small fragments or blast
- Missing progressive hypoxia of lung contusion

Penetrating injuries (fragmentation)

Modern military munitions are designed to produce fragments of a uniform size with a consistent dispersal and injury pattern. Older munitions and IEDs tend to fragment in a random way.

Injury patterns following an explosion depend on protection (combat body armour, vehicle protective armour, intervening objects such as a wall), the trajectory of missiles and the distance from the explosion.

Penetrating wounds from ballistic fragments should be treated as any other penetrating injury, remembering that military wounds are invariably contaminated.

Multiple penetrating wounds require careful assessment to determine which are superficial and which require urgent action to control haemorrhage or repair of deep organs. Ultrasound is useful to examine body cavities in the emergency department, but a single examination does not rule out organ injury.

CT scan or low-dose full body x-ray systems add value to define the fragment path and rule out injury. These may not be available, particularly in field conditions: in this instance repeated physical examination is mandatory.

Some vascular injuries develop arterial venous fistulae that expand slowly and do not become clinically evident for weeks or months after the injury.

Multiple fragments at close range can cause complete obliteration of tissue, resulting in major complex soft tissue wounds. These are managed with initial haemorrhage control, and extensive debridement of debris and devitalized tissue. *Repeat* debridement may be necessary.

The principles of war surgery (also propagated by the International Committee of the Red Cross) are to leave the wound dressings undisturbed for 3–5 days following initial debridement, then surgically reassess and close the wounds if clean (this is *delayed primary closure*). If the patient deteriorates or the wound is offensive it should be reviewed *before* 3–5 days.

For large soft tissue wounds
- Control haemorrhage
- Debride foreign material and dead tissue
- Leave wounds open: primary closure will result in infection

Blunt and crush injury

A clear history of how the patient was injured is the key to guiding the evaluation. There are no special considerations for blunt and crush injuries: treat as conventional injuries. Beware occult blunt injuries because of the distracting nature of penetrating wounds.

Inhalation injury

Treatment is based on the pulmonary symptoms and findings. The symptoms may be progressive, so a period of observation is necessary if inhalation occurred in an enclosed space. Burning plastics, chemicals, furniture, body armour (especially Kevlar®) all give off vapours toxic to the lungs: the presence of these on the patient is not toxic to rescuers.

CHAPTER 6

AUSTERE AND MAJOR INCIDENTS

TRAUMA IN AUSTERE LOCATIONS

Definitions
Definitions of some of the relevant terms are found in Table 6.1.

Expectations in advanced trauma systems
The majority of this book is written from the perspective of people working in advanced trauma systems.

To determine what can be achieved in an austere or remote area to care for the major trauma casualty, a number of factors need to be considered. The aim of this short chapter is not to give all the answers but rather to provide some guidance on these factors and direct the reader to additional resources. The issues discussed are those that have, in the authors' experience, been difficult for people on their first military or non-governmental organization (NGO) deployment to come to terms with.

The care expected for a multiply injured casualty is defined in the box below:

Care pathway for a multiply injured casualty

Emergency services are sent to the scene of the incident
↓
The casualty receives appropriate care
↓
The casualty is taken to a functioning hospital

Although this may appear to be a linear process, it is actually achieved by interaction between a number of systems and their components, including the following.

TABLE 6.1 Definitions	
Austere	*Harsh, severe*
Remote	Out of the way; situated away from the main centres of population
Resource	The means available to achieve an end; a stock or supply that can be drawn on
Infrastructure	The basic structural foundations of a society or enterprise
From The Oxford English Reference Dictionary, 1995	

Communications
- To initiate an Emergency Services response
- To communicate from the incident scene to the hospital
- To coordinate activities in the hospital (e.g. trauma team activation)

The communications systems involved may include radio (HF and VHF) and telephone (landline, satellite or mobile).

Vehicles
- To respond to the scene and carry the casualty
- Vehicles need
  — crew
  — fuel
  — maintenance
  — resupply/replenishment procedures for consumables (dressings, i.v. fluids, drugs) after the call-out

People
This includes pre-hospital personnel (fire, police, ambulance) and in-hospital personnel (doctors, nurses, operating department practitioners, radiographers, laboratory staff, porters, pharmacy, administration support).

To function, the people need to be

- Trained
- Equipped
- Able to reach their place of work (i.e. not prevented by civil disturbance or other threats)

Infrastructure
This includes

- Roads (maintained, lit)
- Utilities (power, water, sewage management, garbage collection)
- Hospitals
  — with functioning utilities
  — with working equipment (CT scanners, anaesthetic machines, sterilizing equipment, ventilators, etc.)
  — with in-date consumables (drugs, fluids, medical gases, blood)
  — with working resupply systems
  — which are maintained (cleaned, repaired)

Clinical expectations and actions are based around these components being in place and working. Protocols, standards and care plans are also based on this. If components are removed or restricted there will be an impact on the ability to provide care.

Restrictions

Working in remote or austere environments means being subject to restrictions. This can mean anything from irregular mail delivery to water rationing. The nature and severity of the restrictions depends on the circumstances. No restriction can be considered in isolation as there will be consequences in other areas.

Some examples are considered below.

Security

Security issues range from petty crime (resulting in loss of equipment and supplies) to being directly threatened. Hostile action may deny access to certain roads or routes, or may even involve the hospital and staff being targeted.

Effects on patient care include

- Non-availability of a resource owing to theft
- Staff unable to cross conflict lines to get to work
- Casualty evacuation from the scene or from hospital being compromised
- If carers are wearing protective equipment such as helmets and body armour they will become fatigued more quickly than usual

Health and hygiene

If the local water supply is poor and diarrhoeal diseases are prevalent, and other endemic diseases threaten the population, then major trauma care will assume a low priority compared with managing these. A balance has to be managed between *population* health needs and an *individual's* health needs.

Poor health infrastructure may impact on the screening, storage and availability of donated blood. Surgical teams need to adjust their blood policies accordingly.

If carers are debilitated by disease or by preventative measures (such as antimalarials), then their ability to manage trauma patients may be decreased.

Infrastructure

Infrastructure was briefly mentioned above. Patient care in a modern trauma system relies heavily on having power, light and water.

At The Pristina University Hospital during the Kosovo conflict of 1999, the mortality rate for ventilated patients was 100%. One of the main factors was power cuts. There were back supplies but the individual tasked to turn on the generators only worked limited hours

Expectations in the field

Understanding restrictions helps to shape expectations for remote and austere environments.

The standard of care can be very high in remote and austere locations. For example, some military medical services can project teams capable of body cavity surgery and appropriate intensive care into very difficult and remote environments. This is, however, heavy on resources.

By contrast, the standards of care can be very low in large urban areas in times of conflict or disaster. An example might be a town or city where the medical infrastructure has been damaged or targeted by combatants.

For trauma care, an additional requirement is to understand likely *mechanisms of injury.* One mechanism of conflict-related injury is shown in Table 6.2. Some of the typical characteristics of war wounds are that they are

- Contaminated
- Contain devitalized tissue
- Affect more than one body cavity
- Often involve multiple injuries
- 75% affect the limbs
- Often present late

A trauma team working in an advanced system would expect patients with these injuries to undergo surgery with blood transfusion, if needed, followed by intensive care and ventilation, if required.

In a resource-limited environment, surgery may need to be performed without blood, and postoperative ventilation may not be available. Current International Committee of the Red Cross (ICRC) protocols do not include postoperative ventilation, and so anaesthetic and surgical techniques need to be adapted accordingly.

As individuals experienced in NGO deployments and war surgery are aware, cavity surgery *can* be performed in the absence of muscle relaxation using ketamine anaesthesia and/or regional

TABLE 6. 2 Mechanisms of injury in antipersonnel mine injury	
Type 1	Traumatic amputation of the lower limb from standing on a mine
Type 2	Random fragment injuries from a mine exploding near a victim
Type 3	Upper limb and facial injuries occurring as a result of handling a mine

anaesthetic techniques. The operating conditions and patient safety are suboptimal compared to that obtained by a trained anaesthetist providing anaesthesia with muscle relaxation.

Coupland (1994) has clearly described how, in the absence of competent surgical facilities, it is better to manage some abdominal injuries conservatively with fluid and antibiotics rather than poorly performed surgery.

Triage
When demand for resources outstrips supply then triage is necessary.

- In advanced trauma systems triage is used to identify the most severely injured so they can be treated first
- In resource-limited situations triage may be needed to identify and then exclude these casualties so that efforts can be concentrated on those with a better chance of survival

Levels of care and sustainability
In every health system there are cut-off points beyond which it is not appropriate to continue to provide resuscitative care. This raises difficult ethical issues.

The decision will be made at different points in different systems and will be influenced by constraints such as resources, culture, money and the nature of the illness/injury. It is useful to consider what levels of care can realistically be provided in a particular situation.

Levels of care
- Basic first aid
  — simple airway manoeuvres/adjuncts, casualty positioning to prevent aspiration, external haemorrhage control, limb splintage and analgesia
- Advanced resuscitation
  — advanced life support (ALS), advanced trauma life support® (ATLS®), British Army trauma life support® (BATLS®)
  — to include invasive procedures such as surgical airways, i.v. access and chest drainage
- Anaesthesia
  — safe rapid sequence induction of anaesthesia and endotracheal intubation using anaesthetic drugs
- The ability to perform safe surgery
- The ability to maintain anaesthesia, endotracheal intubation and muscle relaxation
  — to allow safe *cavity* surgery

- Competent postoperative care
  — including the ability to manage the patient needing
  ventilation and invasive monitoring

Sustainability
Having decided the level of care that can be provided consider

- How long can this be sustained?
- Will this time period allow this patient to recover or be
  evacuated?
- Will this decrease our ability to care for other patients?
- Would a less extensive procedure or course of action be better?
- Would holding procedures (antibiotics, analgesia, fluid and
  nutrition) be better than attempting surgery?

Summary
Providing care in resource-limited environments is a balance of
logistic and clinical issues. These need to be worked through at
an early stage. These are very difficult problems and there are not
answers to fit every situation.

Reading biographies and autobiographies from people
who have worked in these areas can be a very helpful way of
understanding the processes and decisions involved.

REFERENCE

Coupland R M 1994 Epidemiological approach to the surgical management
of the casualties of war. British Medical Journal 308:1693–1697

FURTHER READING

System assessment and general background reading
Hospitals for war wounded 1998. ICRC, Geneva
Keuhl A (ed.) 1994 Prehospital systems and medical oversight (2nd edn).
Mosby–Year Book, St Louis
Perrin P 1996 Handbook on war and public health. ICRC Geneva
Redmond A, Mahoney P F, Ryan J M, Macnab C 2006 ABC of conflict and
disaster. Blackwell Publishing, Oxford

First aid
British Red Cross 2003 Practical first aid. Dorling Kindersley, London
Molde A, Navein J, Coupland R 2001 Care in the field for victims of
weapons of war. ICRC, Geneva

Ballistics and war surgery

Husum, H, Ang S C, Fosse E 1995 War surgery field manual. Third world
network, Penang
Husum, H, Gilbert M, Wisborg T 2000 Save lives, save limbs. Third world
network, Penang
Mahoney P, Ryan J M, Brooks A, Schwab W (eds) 2005 Ballistic trauma, 2nd
edn. Springer Verlag, London
Surgery for victims of war, 3rd edn 1998 ICRC, Geneva

Security

Lloyd Roberts D 1999 Staying alive: safety and security guidelines for
humanitarian volunteers in conflict areas. ICRC, Geneva

Biography/autobiography

Baiev K 2003 The Oath. Simon & Shuster, London
Cutting P 1988 Children of the siege. Pan Books, London
Fink S 2003 War hospital. Public affairs, New York
Giannou C 1991 Besieged. Bloomsbury, London
Kaplan J 2001 The dressing station. Picador, London

ANNEX: CHAIN OF CARE

In the UK and most developed countries, telephoning an
emergency access number triggers an emergency medical services
response.

This is not the case in all countries and is unlikely in austere or
post-conflict environments.

The response to an accident can be seen as a chain of events.

After an accident someone needs to recognize that it has
happened, give first aid and call for help. The 'help' needs to
be dispatched and to be able to find the incident. The people
responding require a set of skills and suitable equipment. They
need to be able to take the casualty to a suitable destination.

In remote/austere environments consider

- How to get help
  — telephone (landline/mobile/satellite) or radio
  — are these working?
  — what help is needed?
- How far away is the help?
- How will the help find the casualty?
- Are they coming by ground vehicle or by air?
  — if air: is it fixed wing or rotary?
  — what landing site is needed?
- What is the level of training of the team responding?

- Where will they take the casualty?
  Regarding medical facilities consider
- Who runs them?
  — host nation, local civil or military
  — foreign military (to the country concerned: e.g. UN, NATO)
  — aid agency
  — private company
- What is their actual capability?
  — reliability of power, water, light; standards of hygiene, safety of blood supplies, training of staff, availability of medicines, dressings, etc.
- How are they accessed?
  — will they treat everyone? Treat insured people only? Treat military only? Treat civilians only? Is a particular ethnic or social group at risk in the hospital?

MAJOR INCIDENTS

Background

For the health service, a major incident is one in which the location, number, severity or type of live casualties requires extraordinary resources.

The priorities set out in the Major Incident Medical Management and Support (MIMMS) guidelines, and used both at the scene and at the hospital are

- Command and control
- Safety
- Communication
- Assessment
- Triage
- Treatment
- Transfer

Hospital staff may, as part of an immediate care scheme or as members of a Medical Emergency Response Incident Team (MERIT), be sent to the scene of an incident. To do this safely and effectively requires special training. Further information on this can be found from the British Association for Immediate Care (www.basics.org.uk) and the Faculty of PreHospital Care at the Royal College of Surgeons in Edinburgh (www.rcsed.ac.uk, then follow link to Faculty) 7 January 2007

This chapter is aimed at the hospital staff remaining in their base hospital and receiving casualties from an incident.

Preparation

All hospitals in the UK with a 24-h emergency department are required to have a major incident plan. This sets out how the hospital will operate during a major incident and allocates additional roles and duties. In addition, each hospital must have an Emergency Planning Officer responsible for the plan and for exercising the response regularly.

Plans should have a *generic component*, which all staff must read, and *action cards* for key individuals. Good plans are simple and keep most staff doing close to their normal job.

Before a major incident is declared
- Read the generic part of your hospital plan and your action card
- Understand how you will be informed on and off duty
- Be sure where you are to report to
- Confirm your role within the plan
- Take part in table-top exercises and full scale rehearsals

Response

The hospital response is directed by the Hospital Control Team, which comprises

- Medical coordinator: a consultant (specialty is hospital-dependent)
- Senior manager
- Senior nurse
- Emergency medicine consultant

The roles of the junior doctor are likely to be:

- On-duty, inform other members of your team and call in other teams
- Off-duty, attend the staff reporting area and await tasking to wards/theatres or to treatment/transport teams in the emergency department

Practically, 'extraordinary resources' for a hospital means

- Additional staff called in
- Additional areas used to receive patients

Both these will be sources of confusion unless personnel understand

- Where to report

- That they must wait there for tasking rather than going straight to the emergency department
- What additional areas are being used
- Where these are
- How patients will get there: '*Casualty flow*'

Triage

Triage means to *sieve* or to *sort* into categories. In a major incident, patients are given priorities for *treatment, investigation* and *surgery*.

Simple triage systems are used at the scene and on arrival at hospital.

Decisions on the order of surgery are more difficult and will depend on the surgeons and theatres available as well as the patients. A senior surgeon must be responsible for these.

Although the Emergency Services at the scene will perform triage and attempt to direct casualties to the appropriate hospital, patients who are not trapped will usually leave the scene first. They may have less severe injuries than those who are trapped. People with minor injuries will 'self-evacuate' and find their own way to hospital. All casualties are assessed or reassessed on arrival at hospital and directed to the correct area. This ensures the best use of emergency department resources.

Patient tracking and documentation

A large number of patients may arrive in a short period of time. In addition, relatives and friends will be trying to find out where a casualty has been taken. The police will send a documentation team to each receiving hospital to help, but systems for patient tracking and rapid documentation must be set up in advance.

Pre-packed sets of documents should be available at the initial triage point. Each set should

- Be labelled with a major incident patient number
- Contain a wrist band with that same number
- A wrist band is put on each patient at triage
- The patient number and initial triage category can then be recorded in a register and on the tracking system
- Further patient movements are fed back to the control team using tracer forms

Each document set should include investigation forms, as manual ordering of tests will usually be necessary because patients will often not be registered onto the computer system fast enough.

Agreement should have been reached with the laboratory services that investigations may be ordered using only the major incident number.

A single receiving ward should also be used so that patients are not spread throughout the hospital.

REFERENCE

The Oxford English Reference Dictionary 1995 Oxford University Press, Oxford

FURTHER READING

Major incident medical management and support (MIMMS) instructors manual, 2nd edn. 2002 London, BMJ Books
UK Department of Health Guidance:
http://www.dh.gov.uk/PolicyandGuidance/EmergencyPlanning/fs/en 7 January 2007

CHAPTER 7

ANAESTHESIA AND ANALGESIA

GENERAL ANAESTHESIA AND SURGERY

General anaesthesia may be initiated in the emergency department when it is clear that an unstable patient is going to require immediate surgery. On occasions, selective procedures for haemorrhage control will be undertaken in the emergency department, e.g. external fixation of pelvic fractures. In such situations, anaesthesia and damage control surgery become an integral part of the patient's resuscitation.

In practice, general anaesthesia is used in the emergency department during resuscitation to achieve definitive airway control by endotracheal intubation. This is performed with a rapid sequence induction (RSI) in which i.v. anaesthetic agents are given with the fast but short-acting muscle relaxant suxamethonium.

The procedure requires specialized training and equipment because of the attendant difficulties; these include unstable shocked patients with unknown or unstable cervical spine status with or without full stomachs, and decreased consciousness levels. The whole process is equipment- and labour-intensive, not least because there must be the means to manage complications, e.g. failure to intubate. Once definite airway control is assured, anaesthesia and muscle relaxation can be maintained using infusions or long-acting drugs.

ANAESTHESIA CHECKLIST

No pocketbook is a substitute for clinical experience: the following is a checklist to aid the trained anaesthesia provider.

- <C>Catastrophic haemorrhage is everyone's concern. Check that sources of major bleeding have been identified and, where possible, dealt with
- Communicate with the team: people need to know that you are about to perform a RSI. Your assistants need to know exactly what is expected of them, e.g. preoxygenation, applying immobilization, giving cricoid pressure, etc.
- Collar: this makes laryngoscopy difficult. Substitute collar and other devices for manual in-line immobilization (the collar can just be opened rather than taken off completely)
- Critical circulation: think large-bore i.v. access
  — consider siting subclavian lines on the same side as the chest drain (if one is in situ)
  — do not site extremity lines distal to injuries: the drugs and fluid are likely to leak out

— in burns consider fixing lines with surgical staples
— be aware of vascular injury when siting lines: will the chosen line site impede surgical access or deny use of a vessel as a graft?

A: Anticipate a difficult airway in trauma. Options include: RSI with the ability to go to a surgical airway if endotracheal intubation is not possible; inhalation induction; awake fibreoptic intubation in selected patients

Think: introducer, bougie, smaller endotracheal tube

B: Remember positive pressure ventilation may convert a simple pneumothorax to a tension pneumothorax. Look for this

C: *Think* circulation: what have induction and intubation done to the blood pressure and cardiac rhythm? Does the patient need fluids? Does the patient need inotropes?

D: Induction agents wear off. What does the patient need to maintain anaesthesia?

E: Now is the opportunity for splinting painful extremities, checking other injuries and preparing to move to the CT scanner, the operating theatre or the ICU

DEFG: Don't ever forget glucose: check that blood sugar has been measured

Anaesthetic induction agent: ketamine

Although several i.v. anaesthetic induction agents are available, ketamine has some particular advantages in trauma. Ketamine produces dissociative anaesthesia. This is a unique pharmacological state characterized by selective suppression of cortical and brainstem function, associated in this case with intense surgical analgesia. Ketamine given intravenously (1–2 mg/kg over 60 s) normally produces some 10 min of anaesthesia. An intramuscular (i.m.) dose of 10 mg/kg should, after 5–10 min, produce 12–25 min of surgical anaesthesia.

Ketamine's action on the sympathetic nervous system produces tachycardia and hypertension. Blood pressure is usually maintained on induction of anaesthesia, which makes it a good choice in shocked patients. Given in smaller doses (less than 1 mg/kg), ketamine is an excellent analgesic, which makes it useful in the emergency department for moving, or performing otherwise painful procedures on, injured patients. When using ketamine, the upper airway reflexes remain more competent than with other sedative agents, but airway competence and protection cannot be assumed. Salivation increases after ketamine, and suction may be required.

Respiratory depression is not usually a problem, although caution is necessary when narcotics or sedatives have been given.

Muscular relaxation is not pronounced and muscle tone may increase.

Ketamine can cause abrupt increases in intracranial pressure (ICP) in patients with intracranial pathology unless blood carbon dioxide levels are controlled by artificial ventilation.

Recovery from ketamine anaesthesia alone can be associated with distressing emergence phenomena. These can be prevented or obtunded with small doses of short-acting i.v. benzodiazepines.

ANALGESIA IN THE EMERGENCY DEPARTMENT

Background
- Resuscitation comes before attempts at pain relief
  — <C>ABC corrects hypoxia and hypovolaemic shock
- Once life-threatening injuries have been identified and treated, the relief of pain will further assist in relieving the pathophysiology of injury

Treatment principles
Pain is treated using the '3 Ps'

- Psychology: humanitarian reassurance
- Physical methods: splintage, traction and reduction of fractures, cooling of burns
- Pharmacology: drugs, including systemic analgesics, local and general anaesthesia

Pain control is superior when drugs and techniques are combined to influence the pain pathways at different sites: 'multimodal' therapy.

This approach maximizes the advantages of each agent while minimizing unwanted side effects by reducing the doses of individual drugs. This helps to maintain a normal physiological state. Examples are: (a) a sprained ankle—appropriate bandaging and support, supplemented with regular oral analgesics; (b) a fractured femur—initial control with i.v. morphine and a femoral nerve block to allow formal reduction and splintage.

Systemic analgesia
Drugs can be administered by a number of routes. The choice of route will depend on how the drug is formulated and the condition of the casualty.

Oral analgesia

Oral analgesics are used in the less seriously injured. In treating musculoskeletal and soft tissue injuries the combined use of simple analgesics with non-steroidal anti-inflammatories (NSAIDs) is usually very effective.

After serious injury, gastric emptying and gut motility are likely to be delayed and patients are prone to vomiting, so oral treatment is not normally an initial option.

Intramuscular injection

Intramuscular injection of drugs may be necessary when personnel lack cannulation skills, resources are limited, or casualties present in large numbers.

Intramuscular injection has a number of limitations. Onset of drug action is unpredictable and will be delayed in the shocked and cold patient. Subsequent fluid resuscitation and rewarming following an i.m. injection can result in the drug being rapidly 'washed' out of the muscle into the circulation. This in turn may produce cardiovascular and respiratory depression.

Intravenous injection

Intravenous injection provides a faster onset of analgesia and is best done by giving small amounts of the drug slowly through an i.v. cannula and monitoring the patient's response.

INDIVIDUAL PHARMACOLOGY AND TECHNIQUES

Non-opioid analgesics

Paracetamol has a good analgesic action and, unlike aspirin, causes minimal gastric irritation. For adults, between 500 mg and 1 g is taken up to four times a day. With the correct dosage other side effects are rare. Paracetamol is dangerous in overdose and can cause fatal liver damage.

Non-steroidal anti-inflammatory drugs (NSAIDs)

This group of drugs, which includes ibuprofen, diclofenac and ketorolac, is used to treat musculoskeletal and postoperative pain. They have been shown to have opioid-sparing effects. A range of drugs is available, but they differ in terms of recommended dosage, dosage interval, licensed route of administration and severity of side effects.

There are also a number of disadvantages and limitations to the use of NSAIDs

- They can inhibit platelet aggregation and prolong bleeding time, resulting in an increase in bleeding during surgery
- Postoperative haemorrhage has also been reported
- They have been implicated in acute renal failure, particularly in patients with diminished renal perfusion
- They may exacerbate asthma (very rare in the author's experience), cause gastric irritation, and are often avoided in aspirin-sensitive people

These concerns limit their initial use in major injury associated with haemorrhage and shock.

Opioid analgesics

These drugs remain the gold standard by which other analgesic agents are judged, particularly for treating severe visceral pain. Many synthetic and semisynthetic drugs are available, but certain comments are relevant to all opioids

- In severe pain small incremental doses should, where possible, be administered by the i.v. route, and patient response closely observed both to assess pain relief and check for adverse effects (particularly for signs of respiratory depression)
- The opiate antagonist naloxone must always be available, as should be the facilities for advanced airway management
- Antiemetics will frequently be necessary when opioids have been used
- Certain of these drugs are controlled and are subject to the Misuse of Drugs Regulations

The above disadvantages have been partially offset by certain synthetic opioids such as nalbuphine and tramadol. These are characterized by a low potential for respiratory depression and addiction.

Morphine

This is the standard narcotic analgesic against which all other opioids should be assessed. Its classic actions of analgesia with euphoria (and ultimately physical dependence) and respiratory depression depend upon an agonist (positive) action upon CNS opioid receptors. These effects are reversible with the opiate antagonist naloxone. A 1 mg/ml solution can be used to provide an adult bolus injection of between 2 and 5 mg, followed by 1-mg increments according to patient response. Intravenous analgesia may be expected in some 5–10 minutes. Cardiovascular effects include a lowering of blood pressure from systemic vasodilatation following histamine release.

Morphine is generally avoided in the initial management of head injuries, as hypercapnia may occur and pupillary assessment during neurological examination may become more difficult.

Nalbuphine
This is an injectable (subcutaneous, i.m. or i.v.) synthetic opioid characterized by its minimal abuse potential. A dose of 10–20 mg is given 3–6-hourly as necessary. Its analgesic effect and degree of respiratory depression are stated to be similar to morphine, while nausea and vomiting may be less. Reports of clinical effect in hospital are varied, but pre-hospital use is reported to be safe and effective.

Tramadol
This is another synthetic weak opioid given by the oral, i.v. or i.m. route. A dose of 50–100 mg is given 6-hourly, although up to 400 mg is permissible as a single bolus. Significant opioid side effects are infrequent, although some patients will hallucinate and seizures have also been recorded.

Codeine phosphate
This is an opioid with good analgesic activity. A dose of 30–60 mg is given orally or intramuscularly 4–6-hourly, up to a maximum of 240 mg a day. Constipation and drowsiness may occasionally be problems, particularly with prolonged use in the elderly.

The influence of opioids given pre-hospital
Theoretically, undesirable interactions are possible if opioids given in hospital interact with synthetic opioids given earlier. This is because of selective effects on the different types of opioid receptors that occur in the CNS. In practice such antagonism is rare but, before administering any drug in hospital, it must never be forgotten that any combination of CNS depressants (head injury, alcohol, sedatives, analgesics) must be expected to act in an additive fashion, with a predictable effect on level of consciousness.

Inhalational analgesia
Pre-mixed 50:50 nitrous oxide and oxygen (Entonox®) has been a traditional analgesic in UK emergency and obstetric practice for over 50 years. Its popularity rests on its ease of administration and safety. The mixture is provided from on-demand valved cylinders and administered via a mask or mouthpiece. The delivery should be patient-controlled so that, in the unlikely event of impending unconsciousness, the situation is corrected as the patient releases the mouthpiece.

Analgesia will peak some 2–5 min after inhalation and this fact needs to be respected when Entonox® is used to assist painful procedures. Entonox® is contraindicated in decompression illness as it will expand gas bubbles that are present. It is also contraindicated in pneumothorax, unless there is a functioning chest drain in situ.

Nitrous oxide diffuses out of the bloodstream into gas-filled cavities (and bubbles) faster than nitrogen can be removed, causing an increase in pressure and volume within these spaces.

Theoretically, similar considerations apply to air collections within the cranial cavity of head-injured patients. In practice the short-term use of Entonox® should be safe for a casualty with mild concussion and pain from other injuries.

Local anaesthesia

The use of local anaesthetic techniques can provide safe and effective analgesia for some acute trauma problems. In the emergency department local anaesthesia is most commonly used for.

- Infiltration: direct injection of local anaesthetic into skin and subcutaneous tissues for wound exploration and suturing, or to assist procedures such as chest drain insertion
- Individual nerve blocks: those selected are specific nerve blocks which can be performed quickly and safely
  — femoral nerve block: this may be used to assist splinting or movement of an injured leg during extrication. A 3-cm, 23-gauge needle will be sufficient for non-obese patients. The nerve is frequently more superficial (1–1.5 cm depth) than taught in some trauma skills courses. As a quick onset analgesia is required, lidocaine (lignocaine) is a suitable anaesthetic, and bilateral blocks are permissible within the maximum safe doses (MSD). The local anaesthetic should be deposited in a fan-shaped distribution so as to accommodate variable distances of the nerve lateral to the femoral artery. Careful aspiration prior to and during deposition will ensure that inadvertent vascular injection does not occur
  — peripheral hand blocks: ring blocks of digits or single nerve blocks at the wrist are of value when assessing hand injuries
  — haematoma blocks: direct injection of a fracture haematoma is useful for certain limb fractures, particularly at the wrist. There is a role for these blocks when dealing with large numbers of casualties and in elderly or frail patients. Attention to sterile technique is important to avoid

introducing infection into the haematoma, and
adrenaline-containing solutions should be avoided
— i.v. regional anaesthesia (Biers block): this allows anaesthesia
by i.v. injection of local anaesthetic into a limb which has
been exsanguinated by a tourniquet. It used to be a very
popular emergency department technique, but deaths have
occurred and its safety is dependent upon the use of a
double tourniquet technique and the absolute avoidance of
bupivacaine (see below).

Local anaesthetic safety

Local anaesthetic safety is important. The potential danger will
vary according to the technique proposed, patient condition and
the agent selected.

Safety is maximized by

- Prior placement of an i.v. cannula to permit resuscitation
- Ensuring unintended intravascular injection of local anaesthetic
  does not occur
- Respecting the recommended MSD and, where practical,
  avoiding the use of solutions containing adrenaline (used to
  prolong the duration of action of the local anaesthetic) so that
  systemic absorption of adrenaline or injection into areas of
  vascular compromise cannot occur

The MSDs quoted below refer to the use of large volumes for
infiltration and specific nerve blocks, where there is no intended
direct or indirect vascular or cerebrospinal fluid injection.

Local anaesthetic agents

- Lidocaine (lignocaine): a rapid-acting synthetic amide available
  in 0.5, 1 or 2% concentrations with or without adrenaline
  (1:200 000 = final concentration of 5 micrograms of adrenaline
  per millilitre). The MSD is 4 mg/kg without adrenaline and
  6 mg/kg with adrenaline. 1–2% solutions are suitable for most
  infiltration and nerve block techniques. Analgesia will persist for
  2–4 h
- Prilocaine: similar in efficacy and safety to lidocaine, but its
  MSD permits safe administration of up to 40 ml of a 0.5%
  solution. This makes it the agent of choice for Biers block
- Bupivacaine: a long-acting amide with a slow onset of action. It
  is available in 0.125, 0.25, 0.5 and 0.75% concentrations with or
  without adrenaline. The MSD is 2 mg/kg. Bupivacaine is widely
  used in hospital practice, but the advantage it affords by being

long-acting (up to 6–8 h) must be balanced against its toxicity. Cardiorespiratory collapse following accidental i.v. injection of bupivacaine may prove fatally resistant to resuscitation. Bupivacaine occurs as a racemic mixture and separation of its L-isomer is now available as this agent has a significantly less cardiotoxic profile

 Bupivacaine is not suitable for Biers block

- Ropivacaine: this is another newer development following the concerns of cardiotoxicity of bupivacaine. It has a similar analgesia profile to racemic bupivacaine but, like the L-isomer of bupivacaine, is less cardiotoxic

FURTHER READING

British National Formulary September 2006 BMJ Publishing Group, London

CHAPTER 8

SCORING SYSTEMS

INJURY SEVERITY SCORING

Background

There are three types of injury scoring: anatomical, physiological and combined. Whilst this list is not exhaustive, it includes the most validated and common systems currently in use. Knowledge and understanding of these scores is useful to interpret the trauma literature accurately, decipher operative reports, and comprehend methods of predicting patient outcome, including death and complications. For further scoring systems refer to the further reading list.

SCORING SYSTEMS

Anatomical
- Abbreviated injury scale (AIS)
- Injury severity score (ISS)
- New injury severity score (NISS)
- Penetrating abdominal trauma index (PATI)
- Organ injury scale (OIS)
- Mangled extremity score (MES)

Physiological
- Glasgow coma score (GCS)
- Trauma score (TS)
- Revised trauma score (RTS)

Combined
- Trauma and injury severity score (TRISS)

Anatomical injury severity scoring

Abbreviated injury scale

The AIS was developed by the Association for the Advancement of Automotive Medicine in 1969 and is the most widely used anatomical injury severity scale in the world. It was originally developed for use by crash investigators to standardize data on the frequency and severity of motor vehicle-related injuries. It is now universally accepted and used to calculate the ISS and the NISS. Its use has also been extended to epidemiological research, studies to predict survival probability, patient outcome evaluation and healthcare systems research. It is likely to remain the basic system to assess overall injury severity.

Injuries are ranked on a scale of 1–6, with 1 being minor, 5 severe and 6 an unsurvivable injury (Table 8.1). This represents the 'threat to life' associated with an injury. These scores are incorporated into an AIS code for each specific injury and are used to calculate the injury severity score.

The injury severity score

The ISS is an anatomical scoring system that provides an overall score for patients with multiple injuries. Each injury is assigned an AIS score and is allocated to one of six body regions. Only the highest AIS score in each body region is used. The three most severely injured body regions have their score squared and added together to produce the ISS score, i.e. $X^2 + Y^2 + Z^2 = $ total.

Calculation of the injury severity score (Table 8.2)

- Allocate injuries to a body region. to determine a patient's ISS, a score is allocated to each of the patient's injuries; only one score may be taken from each of the six body regions
  — head or neck (including cervical spine)
  — face
  — chest (including thoracic spine)
  — abdominal or pelvic contents (including lumbar spine)
  — extremities or pelvic girdle
  — external (lacerations, contusions, abrasions and burns)
- Allocate a code and AIS score to each injury: a regularly updated (most recently in 2005) comprehensive coding book is used to allocate codes and determine the ISS. At the end of each code is a decimal point; for example, the code for a cerebral contusion is 140604.3, thus the AIS score is 3. The AIS scores range from 1 to 6, as described in Table 8.1.

TABLE 8.1 Abbreviated injury scale severity scores	
AIS score	*Injury*
1	Minor
2	Moderate
3	Serious
4	Severe
5	Critical
6	Unsurvivable

TABLE 8.2 Calculation of the injury severity score (ISS)				
Body region	Injury	AIS code	Highest AIS	AIS²
Head/neck	Small subdural haemorrhage Odontoid (dens) fracture	140652.4 650228.3	4	16
Face	Zygoma fracture	251800.2	2	
Chest	Sternum fracture	450802.2	2	
Abdomen	Grade 3 liver laceration	541824.3	3	9
Extremities	Open—humerus fracture	752604.3	3	9
External	Multiple abrasions	910200.1	1	
AIS, abbreviated injury scale				

Injury severity score groups

Patients are commonly grouped according to their ISS to allow for more valid comparisons between patient groups. An ISS score below 9 usually represents a minor injury, a score between 9 and 15 a moderate injury, and one greater than 15 a severe injury. ISS allows for comparisons of outcomes between different hospitals and trauma systems, and facilitates a more rational allocation of resources and manpower, since injury severity is a more accurate predictor of the quantity and intensity of care that a trauma centre is likely to provide than are simple patient numbers.

Is the injury severity score really indicative of injury severity?

As the patient may have three serious scores in one body region, and only one score is permitted to calculate the ISS, the true severity of patient injury may not always be represented. This often occurs in patients with multiple long bone injuries, who are only able to have one extremity injury included in the ISS calculation. Despite these concerns, ISS remains the most widely used injury severity scoring system, largely because no other method has been found that both increases the accuracy of mortality predictions and justifies an industry-wide switch to a new system.

New injury severity score

In 1997, Osler et al described the NISS, which enables the sum of the squares of the AIS scores of a patient's three most severe

TABLE 8.3 Calculation of the injury severity score (ISS) vs. the new injury severity score (NISS)

Body region	Injury	AIS code	Highest AIS	AIS^2 for ISS	AIS^2 for NISS
Head/neck	Skull (linear)	150402.2	2	4	
Face	Nose	251002.1	1		
Chest	Rib (×1)	450212.1	1	1	
Abdomen	No injury				
Extremities	Open— humerus comminuted	752604.3	3	9	9
	Radius	752804.3	3		9
	Femur	851800.3	3		9
	Pubic ramus	852600.2			
External	Multiple abrasions	910200.1	1		
				ISS = 14	NISS = 27

Note the large difference in score

injuries, regardless of body region (Table 8.3). They (see Further reading) demonstrated that the NISS was more predictive of outcome than the ISS.

Penetrating abdominal trauma index
This scoring system was initially developed in 1981 by Moore and colleagues in Denver, USA, and was subsequently revised in 1990 (Borlase et al, 1990). At laparotomy, a severity score is assigned to each organ injury based on a set of criteria, and a cumulative abdominal trauma index is then derived by adding each organ score. The risk of major septic complications increases exponentially with an ATI score above 25. The PATI has been shown by other investigators to be useful in calculating the risk of septic complications after penetrating abdominal injury.

Organ injury scale
The OIS was developed by the Organ Injury Scaling Committee of the American Association for the Surgery of Trauma (AAST website). Originally convened in 1987, these scoring systems are modified and updated as deemed appropriate. The scale is graded from 1 to 6 for each organ, with 1 being the least severe and 5 the

most severe injury from which the patient may survive. Grade 6 injuries are by definition not salvageable. Scales are available for injuries to the organs/systems listed in Tables 8.4 and 8.5.

Mangled extremity severity score
This is a simple rating scale for lower extremity trauma, based on skeletal/soft tissue damage, limb ischaemia, shock and age. It attempts to predict the necessity of limb amputation. Results of validation studies have been variable.

It is a useful guide for decision-making but is *not absolute* and should be used with caution (Table 8.6).

Physiological injury severity scoring

Glasgow coma score
The GCS is the best known injury scoring system. It is universally accepted as a simple and quick neurological assessment with a range of between 3 and 15. The lower the score, the poorer the neurological status.

Glasgow coma score	
≥13	Mild
12–9	Moderate
≤8	Severe

Note that the phrase 'GCS of 11' is essentially meaningless, and it is important to break the figure down into its components, such as E3V3M5 = GCS 11 (Table 8.7). Three modifiers (S, T and P) are used to describe situations when one or more component of the GCS cannot be accurately described on the numerical scale

TABLE 8.4 Organ injury score body regions		
Cervical vascular	Stomach	Uterus (non-pregnant)
Chest wall	Duodenum	Uterus (pregnant)
Heart	Small bowel	Fallopian tube
Lung	Colon	Ovary
Thoracic vascular	Rectum	Vagina
Diaphragm	Abdominal vascular	Vulva
Spleen	Adrenal organ	Testis
Liver	Kidney	Scrotum
Extrahepatic biliary tree	Ureter	Penis
Pancreas	Bladder	Peripheral vascular organs
Oesophagus	Urethra	

TABLE 8.5 Liver injury scale

Grade	Type of injury	Description	AIS
I	Haematoma	Subcapsular <10% surface area	2
	Laceration	Capsular tear <1 cm parenchymal depth	2
II	Haematoma	Subcapsular 10–50% surface area: intraparenchymal <10 cm in diameter	2
	Laceration	Capsular tear 1–3 cm parenchymal depth, <10 cm in length	
III	Haematoma	Subcapsular >50% surface area of ruptured subcapsular or parenchymal haematoma; intraparenchymal haematoma >10 cm or expanding; 3 cm parenchymal depth	3
	Laceration	Parenchymal disruption involving 25–75% hepatic lobe or one to three Couinaud's segments	4
	Laceration	Parenchymal disruption involving >75% of hepatic lobe or more than three Couinaud's segments within a single lobe	5
	Laceration	Juxtahepatic venous injuries, i.e. retrohepatic vena cava/central major hepatic veins	5
	Vascular	Hepatic avulsion	5

TABLE 8.6 Mangled extremity score	
Criteria	*Score*
Energy of injury	
Low	1
Medium	2
High	3
Massive	4
Limb ischaemia*	
No ischaemia	0
Pulse reduced or absent but perfusion normal	1
Pulseless, paraesthesia, diminished capillary refill	2
Cool, paralysed, insensate, numb	3
Systolic blood pressure	
Normal	0
Transient hypotension	1
Persistent hypotension	2
Age (years)	
<30	0
30–50	1
>50	2

*Ischaemia score doubles when warm ischaemia time >6 h
MESS score of 7 or less: the limb is likely to be salvageable

TABLE 8.7 Adult Glasgow Coma Score		
Eye opening	Spontaneous	4
	To voice	3
	To pain	2
	None	1
	Swollen shut	S
Verbal response	Orientated	5
	Confused	4
	Inappropriate	3
	Incomprehensible	2
	None	1
	Intubated	T
Motor response	Obeys commands	6
	Localizes to pain	5
	Withdraws from pain	4
	Flexion	3
	Extension to pain	2
	None	1
	Paralysed	P
	GCS total score	3–15

A modified version is available for paediatric patients

alone. For example, a patient whose eyes cannot open due to severe periorbital swelling should be assigned an eye component score of '1-S', the 'S' indicating swollen. Similarly, an intubated patient should have the letter 'T' appended (for tube) to the verbal score, and a paralysed patient unable to move extremities should have the motor component appended with the letter 'P'.

Trauma score
The TS combines the patient's GCS, systolic blood pressure, capillary refill and respiratory effort, producing a score ranging from 1 to 16. Lower scores are associated with higher mortality rates. Whilst the TS is a rapid, easy to calculate physiological score and has been in use since 1981, in reality it is not widely used in the pre-hospital or resuscitative phase.

Revised trauma score
The RTS was derived from the TS in 1989, and has been shown to be a better predictor of mortality than the TS. The RTS uses only the respiratory rate, systolic blood pressure and GCS. The range is 0–12; once again, lower scores are associated with higher morbidity and poorer outcomes.

Combined injury severity scoring

Trauma and injury severity score
TRISS is based on regression equations that combine the age, anatomical (ISS) and physiological scores (RTS) of the patient to predict patient survival. For example, a patient with blunt trauma aged 80 years with an ISS of 35 and an RTS of 8 has a probability of survival of 79.5%. TRISS does not indicate at what level of function they would survive; nor does it take into account multiple injuries in one body region or pre-existing conditions, such as heart disease. It has been shown to give a relatively accurate account of whether the patient has a greater or less than 50% chance of survival.

Summary
Injury scoring is an evolving field that, to date, provides a good baseline for retrospective comparison with other centres, an indicator of patient outcomes, a tool for research and a rough guide to predicting patient survival. Research into identifying more accurate injury scoring systems is ongoing and continues to improve. Until the time that simple and accurate predictors exist, injury scoring in the immediate clinical assessment scenario is likely to remain an adjunct to the clinician's skills.

REFERENCES

Borlase B C, Moore E E, Moore F A 1990 The abdominal trauma index—a critical reassessment and validation. The Journal of Trauma 30(11):1340–1344

Osler T, Baker S P, Long W 1997 A modification of the injury severity score that both improves accuracy and simplifies scoring. Journal of Trauma 43(6):922–926

Organ Injury Scale: http://www.aast.org/injury/injury.html 7 January 2007

FURTHER READING

Baker S P, O'Neill B, Haddon W Jr, Long W B 1974 The injury severity score: a method for describing patients with multiple injuries and evaluating emergency care. Journal of Trauma 14(3):187–196

Borlase B C, Moore E E, Moore F A 1990 The abdominal trauma index—a critical reassessment and validation. Journal of Trauma 30(11):1340–1344

Maurer A, Morris J A 2004 Injury severity scoring. In: Moore E E, Feliciano D V, Mattox K L (eds) Trauma, 5th edn. McGraw-Hill, New York, p 87–93

Web links

Trauma scores/ISS/TRISS
http://www.trauma.org/scores/index.html 7 January 2007

PATI calculator
http://www.medalreg.com/qhc/medal/ch29/29_11/29-11-ver9.php3#result 7 January 2007

Lower limb scores
http://www.rcsed.ac.uk/fellows/lvanrensburg/classification/trauma%20scores/mangled_extremity_scores.htm#Mangled%20Extremity%20Severity%20Score%20(MESS)%20Johansen%201990 7 January 2007

INDEX

MAJOR TRAUMA
INDEX ◀ **303**